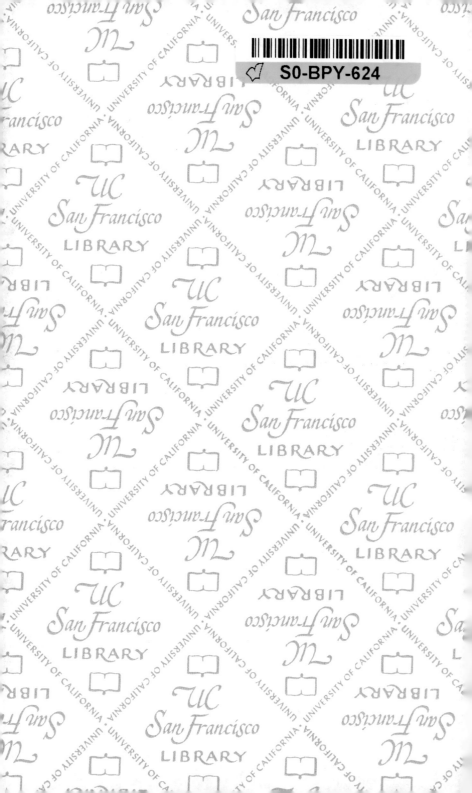

The Spectrum of Pain

by Richard Serjeant

Private Flying
A Man May Drink

Richard Serjeant

The Spectrum of Pain

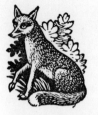

Rupert Hart-Davis   London   1969

© Richard Serjeant 1969
First published in Great Britain 1969
Rupert Hart-Davis Ltd
3 Upper James Street, Golden Square
London W1

Printed in Great Britain by
Ebenezer Baylis and Son Ltd
The Trinity Press
Worcester and London

SBN 246 97465 6

CONTENTS

INTRODUCTION

PAIN is a complex, essential and sometimes terrible part of life. At one time or another nearly all of us encounter severe pain, either in ourselves or in others, and the experience usually has a powerful psychological impact, often leading to speculation about why a sensation with such awful potentialities should have a place in Nature – a question that worries some people very much, to the extent of seeking some rational explanation that will be valid in all circumstances. They find instead many widely differing views, depending on the background, personal experiences, training and philosophical outlook of the writer; it is difficult to know what is true and what is false, because so much appears prejudiced or emotionally coloured or unreasonable – and the individual lacks the background of knowledge on which he can form some kind of judgment.

Statements will be found that pain is the vital protective mechanism of the body; that its purpose is to punish sinners; that its endurance is a virtue that will bring great rewards in after-life; that it is an unequivocal evil; that it only exists in the mind, and so can be conquered by right thinking; that it only affects human beings, not animals; that the complete injustice of its distribution proves that God does not exist; that God's inscrutable purpose in devising the endless manifestations of suffering cannot be explained by mere Man.

Clearly all these cannot be true, and some are based on limited viewpoints. In the parts that follow an effort is made to present a number of facts and comments in as wide a field as possible, providing the reader with a basis on which to form his own opinions. What does emerge is the great complexity of the subject, every aspect of it overlapping others to an extent that renders any artificial division into categories and any expressions of opinion open

7

to severe criticism. Inevitably readers will disagree with much of what is said here, and perhaps feel that the finer and more beautiful aspects of Nature have been ignored. The short answer to this is that we are trying to deal with a grim subject, and it needs all the space available. If people are shocked by what they read or dislike the opinions expressed it means at least that they are thinking about these things, and unless there is some hard constructive thinking about certain aspects of pain in the near future I believe the upward trend of Evolution might cease.

In the course of this work I have received help from many sources; the foremost among these are not conscious of having done so – the patients who have passed through my hands and so often displayed remarkable qualities of courage and fortitude in the face of pain. In acknowledging help from other sources, including many friends and colleagues, I must make it clear that they are in no way responsible for the views expressed in this book, which in many cases will be at variance with theirs. My thanks are due to the Superintendent and staff of the British Museum Reading Room; to the Librarian, the British Medical Association; to the National Society for the Prevention of Cruelty to Children; to the Royal Society for the Prevention of Cruelty to Animals; to the Howard League for Penal Reform; to the Librarian, Guy's Hospital; and to the authors of over a hundred books and articles consulted and sometimes quoted. I am grateful to Mr Patrick Moore for personal communications; to Mr George Northcroft, FRCS, for help with the section on Neurosurgery; to Mr Roy Smith, for information about his use of hypnosis in dentistry; to Mr J. B. Morton (Beachcomber) for permission to quote from his inimitable column, and to the Editor of the *Daily Express*; to Mrs Rosemary Rehling for great help in preparing the manuscript; to Mr Peter Barber for his skill and care with the diagrams; to my Publishers for every possible assistance; and to my wife for her wonderful patience, and for help in many ways.

PART ONE

THE PATHWAYS OF PAIN

PAIN takes many forms, but at its simplest is an appreciation of actual or potential harm to the body. The sensation of pain is impossible to define, but attempts to do so are really unnecessary because almost every human being knows what the word implies — some only too well. This undefinable quality is lacking in other sensations that may be acutely unpleasant, such as a disgusting smell or taste, or hunger, or a sound that sets one's teeth on edge; it is often accompanied by worry or fear, yet some sensations that are not intrinsically painful may cause acute terror — like that of being dropped from a height. Under normal conditions one is free from pain, though it does not follow that because there is no pain all is well. The different tissues and organs of the body vary very widely both in their sensitivity and in the kind of pain felt when they are damaged. The experience of pain is uniquely personal and unpleasant, and brings a compelling urge to do something about it.

We shall have to make some assumptions that may appear reasonable enough but are not susceptible of proof. By definition pain is a conscious phenomenon and therefore does not exist in the unconscious state, however this may be caused. We assume that consciousness is rather a late development in evolution and associated with a fairly complex brain. There are reasons for thinking that the more advanced the brain the greater the capacity for feeling pain and, since a limit must be drawn somewhere, it will be assumed that pain as we know it is an experience shared only by the higher mammalian vertebrates, who have very similar nervous systems.

Ordinary experience shows that normally an injury to the skin surface, for example a sharp prick in a finger, is followed by consciousness of pain in the injured part and also by an involuntary jerking of the part away from the noxious agent. At first sight this may appear to be quite a simple matter — you feel a pain in your finger, so you move it away from the cause. In fact the process is very much more complex than this and there are at least two distinct nervous pathways involved, one conveying the pain into consciousness and the other, a faster circuit, causing the 'withdrawal reflex'. Both are of vital importance to us. Close examination shows that in fact the withdrawal reflex is a fundamental one in the animal kingdom and is practically automatic in action, being complete before pain is actually felt.

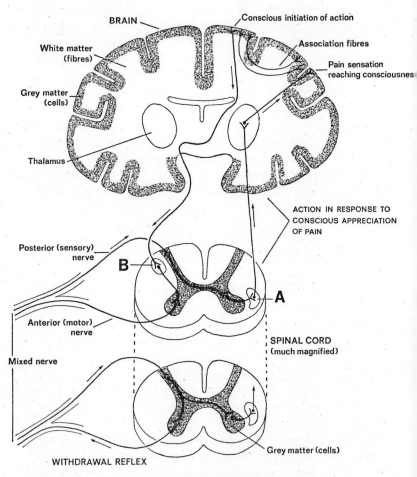

Fig. 1. The Pathways

THE NERVOUS SYSTEM

The body is equipped with a vastly intricate communications system by which information is received from the outside world as well as from its own manifold parts; this information is sorted out by a central mechanism, and *a very small part of it* enters consciousness in the form of sensation, relating the experience to its own accumulated memories and to present situations and the expected future. The central mechanism sends out a stream of messages that result in co-ordinated action by the body's tissues and organs, a *very small part* of this action being consciously directed. These sensations and conscious acts together with our memories, thoughts and dreams, constitute all the life we know — all its excitements and disappointments, achievements and failures, pleasures and pains. It may be objected that this is a grossly materialistic viewpoint, but it is surely true to say that a sentient being can only act rationally on the content of his mind; the origin of such content is of course open to many interpretations.

The nervous system itself is built of millions of microscopic *cells* connected by extensions called *fibres* to each other and to *nerve endings* in the tissues and organs. The fibres are gathered together into cable-like structures constituting the *nerves*, or into the *white matter* of the brain and spinal cord. The *grey matter*, on the outside of the brain and the inside of the spinal cord, mainly consists of closely packed nerve cells and the short connections between them (Figure 1, page 12). Each nerve-cell unit is known as a *neurone*, comprising the cell with its various appendages (Figure 2, page 14). The communications between neurones are indirect, through one-way relays called *synapses*. It will be seen that the possibilities of intercommunication between different parts of the system are enormous indeed, yet the main pathways remain clear and distinct.

Nerves may be compared very roughly with electric wires; they are of two main kinds, the *sensory* nerves that convey information from tissues and organs to the central nervous system (the brain and the spinal cord) and the *motor* nerves conducting the outward impulses that result in action.

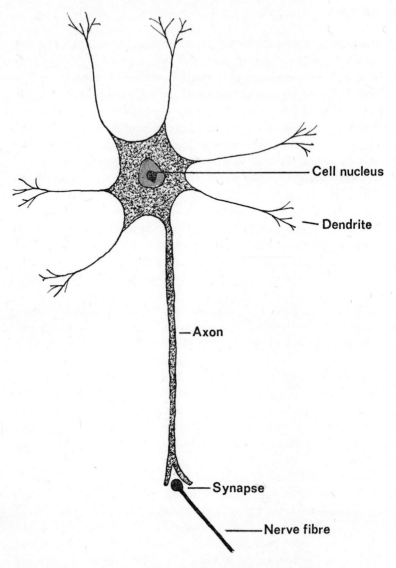

Fig. 2. A Nerve Cell

Sensation

Three main varieties of sensory information are admitted to consciousness — sight, hearing and touch. In addition to these there are
other highly specialized senses such as taste, smell, hunger, position-
sense, balance, temperature-sense and pain. Most of these senses
are distinct, having their own specialized nerve endings in the
appropriate tissues and organs, their own bundle of nerve fibres in
the spinal cord and their own particular terminal area in the brain,
though here very wide overlap occurs because of the enormous
numbers of co-ordinating and association tracts that are necessary.

Of course it does not follow that because the various kinds of
sensation *can* enter consciousness they necessarily do so; we are only
able to perceive a few impressions at any particular time, and while
we can to some extent direct this awareness by an effort of will a
powerful impression will easily over-ride and exclude all others.
Thus a man absorbed in hearing a piece of music finely played may
be unaware of visual stimuli, physical discomforts, hunger and even
other noises, so long as these sensations are not too strong. And the
strongest of all physical sensations is pain.

Pathways

In order to become conscious a sensory impulse must reach the
brain, travelling along nerve fibres and passing through the various
relays on the way. Exactly how nerves transmit this impulse is not
known; but the speed of travel is very much slower than the passage
of electricity along a wire, varying between half a metre and one
hundred metres per second, according to the kind of nerve and its
size. It takes appreciably longer for a message to reach the brain
from the feet than from other parts of the body, and the organs of
acutest awareness (the eyes and ears) lie closest to the brain.

Nerve-endings

The entire surface of the body excepting the eyes, the nails and the natural orifices is covered with skin. This has a very complex structure containing hair-follicles, sweat and other glands, blood-vessels and the sensory nerve-endings. A magnified section through the skin is shown in Figure 3, and a number of these delicate structures can be seen just below the actual skin surface. The

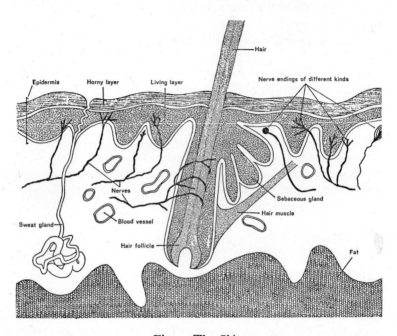

Fig. 3. The Skin

nerve-endings are of several different kinds according to the type of sensation they transmit, so we find special ones for touch, pressure, temperature and for several varieties of pain. A needle entering the skin penetrates the surface and is very likely to stimulate several pain nerve-endings. It is not *certain* to do so because the skin's sensitivity depends partly on the number of nerve-endings crowded into a particular area, and some parts have many more than others. The finger tips are richly supplied with nerves and a prick will usually elicit pain, whereas in the back they are much more scattered, so spots can be found with a needle that do not hurt when pricked. In the Middle Ages these insensitive areas were known as Witch's Spots, and hunted for with zealous cruelty by professional 'witch-finders' armed with long bodkins. The back was of course among the last places to be examined.

The Nature of the Stimulus

If a needle penetrates the skin a minute area of damage is caused; the damage results in impulses which shoot up the nerve itself. What actually causes pain impulses to travel up the nerves? Probably some degree of injury is always involved, however slight, but there seems to be difference between the sudden sharp initial stimulus and the more prolonged pain that follows such an injury. The initial sharp stimulus may perhaps be primarily electrical in nature and all other kinds primarily chemical. The two main kinds of pain can be detected easily – the sudden sharp stab of pain, followed by a slower longer sensation as local chemicals begin to act, and the interval between them is greatest at long distances from the brain – the fingers and toes. (There is a further differentiation between 'fast' and 'slow' pain depending on the actual size of the nerve fibre and its degree of insulation.)

Tissue damage of any kind leads to the immediate release of chemical substances and these initiate a stream of electrical impulses in the nerves. It has actually proved possible to identify certain of these substances, some of which are similar to poisons used by plants and animals for painful stings and bites – some mild, others of extreme violence. The main chemicals concerned are *Histamine*, *5-hydroxytryptamine* and a *plasma polypeptide* – referred to by Samson Wright as the Unholy Trio.[1] It may be of interest to know how these chemicals are tested for their efficacy in stimulating nerve endings. Using human volunteers (usually students, who don't like to say 'no') an irritant chemical such as Cantharides is applied to the skin, resulting in a blister. When this has fully developed the

[1] *Applied Physiology*, Samson Wright. Publication details of all works referred to in the footnotes are given in the Bibliography.

raised epidermis is cut away, releasing the fluid; the raw sensitive base of the blister is exposed complete with its manifold nerve-endings. Various chemical substances can now be applied to the raw surface and their efficacy as pain producers immediately assessed by the victim. It is found that a solution of salt at the same strength as the body's fluid (isotonic saline) causes no pain, whereas weaker (hypotonic) or stronger (hypertonic) saline solutions cause some discomfort. Acids and alkalis cause sharp pain, the Unholy Trio severe pain. The blister fluid itself causes no pain unless it has been in contact with glass, so that if these blisters are aspirated with a glass syringe and the same fluid re-injected acute pain is produced. Cocaine and similar substances cause initial discomfort followed by numbness; the nerve-endings then cease to conduct impulses even when the Unholy Trio are applied and the effect persists for some time. One notable feature of such experiments is the almost complete absence of fear and other kinds of emotional overlay which can profoundly modify reactions in other circumstances.

The distribution of nerves to their own areas of skin is very precise and constant, so that stimulation of one tiny area in the tip of the index finger will always send an impulse up one particular nerve fibre, its identity being maintained in the form of a coded pattern right up to one special area in the brain; by this means we are able to say with some certainty which part of the skin is being damaged – in other words we can *locate* the pain. Pain in other parts of the body may not be at all precisely located, and may indeed be felt in a site remote from the stimulus.

Complex Associations

To state that a prick in the finger results in the feeling of pain there is a gross over-simplication. The original stimulus has to be assessed for severity and duration; it must also be related to all the other sensations arising in the part and elsewhere, as well as to the situation of the whole body, as conveyed by vision and other senses, and by a number of emotional factors. The fact that this particular stimulus was painful is noted, stored in memory systems and related to other similar experiences; and finally the stimulus is related to the action to be taken, either calculated and reasoned or automatic and unconscious. Many of these details are very directly concerned with the functions of pain and will be dealt with later; the point here is that the impulse travelling to the brain is interrupted at many places by relay stations at which branch connections are made with other parts of the nervous system, and therefore with other parts of the body and fields of consciousness.

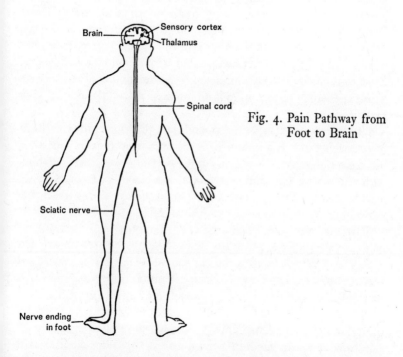

Fig. 4. Pain Pathway from Foot to Brain

A bare-foot man steps on a tin-tack: let us trace the pain impulse from the toe to the brain. This pathway is typical of the entire skin surface as well as some of the deeper sensations.

The initial prick stimulates a number of nerve-endings in the skin of the toe — nerve-endings for the sense of touch as well as those for pain of a 'sharp' type. Impulses travel along a few fibres of the *sciatic* nerve, up the leg and through the pelvis; they enter the vertebral column through special bony canals until they reach the back of the spinal cord, for onward transmission to the brain (Figure 4, page 19).

In the spinal cord the pain impulses reach a mass of cells in the grey matter and are relayed in various directions. One of these brings them into a column of white matter on the opposite side, in which they pass upwards to end in a nucleus in the centre of the brain called the thalamus, with further connections to other parts of the brain. The associated sensation of touch passes to a closely localized part of the surface of the brain known as the *sensory cortex* by which it is accurately localized; but pain fibres have much more diffuse connections with the huge frontal lobes and the parts immediately behind them — areas associated with emotion and memory. Most sensations *can* have emotional components, usually by linkage with experience; but emotion is an intrinsic part of the normal pain experience.

Whether consciousness and thought are functions of the brain or of something else is a matter of hot controversy in some quarters, but from the practical viewpoint it is easier to assume that we think with our brains. Certainly our actions are based on experience, we gain experience through our senses, and sensations must reach the brain in order to become consciously appreciated.

That the burnt child fears the fire may appear self-evident, but consider the process involved. The child touches the pretty red coals and then feels an acute violent pain in his hand. It seems logical that he pulls his hand away because it hurts — in other words that he thinks, 'This hurts. I had better pull my hand away or it will go on hurting'; but in fact this would be much too slow to avoid serious injury and the actual withdrawal from the hot object occurs *before* the pain is appreciated in consciousness, by a mechanism that by-passes the brain altogether. Both the conscious pathway and the withdrawal reflex are shown in Figure 1 (page 12). Let us trace both pathways.

Conscious Action in Response to Pain

We have seen how nerves carrying sensory impulses enter the back of the spinal cord, and after being relayed in the grey matter are transmitted upwards in the white matter at the back and side of the cord. The *front* part of the spinal cord is mainly occupied with cells and fibres connected with action, the *motor* mechanism.

If we take a typical limb nerve like the median nerve for the arm or the huge sciatic nerve in the leg we find that it contains roughly equal numbers of sensory and motor fibres. These two sets of fibres separate just outside the spinal cord; all the sensory fibres enter it near the back and all the motor fibres leave it near the front.

In the *consciously directed* reaction a mixed sensory impulse will enter the cord through the sensory nerve, become relayed in the grey matter and travel up to the brain on the opposite side of the cord in a bundle of fibres somewhere in the region marked A in Figure 1, part of it reaching the sensory cortex; another part of it reaches the region of the thalamus and the sensation is judged to be a painful one. Once the sensation becomes conscious a decision is made about appropriate action and impulses are generated in the motor areas of the brain to carry it out. These impulses, after crossing to the opposite side, travel down the cord in one of the regions marked B, are relayed to the cells in the front part of the grey matter, and thence through the motor nerves to the muscles which will then contract and effect withdrawal – a complex group action of many muscles involving not only contraction of muscles to pull the part away, but simultaneous relaxation of any that would oppose this action.

The Withdrawal Reflex

Now this central 'H' shaped mass of nerve cells in the spinal cord contains millions of delicately balanced connections of its own, and among these is a way of shunting impulses from the sensory nerves directly to the motor nerves at the same level. This means an *automatic* response to certain kinds of stimuli, notably the harmful ones. Again consider the child touching the red-hot coal; the pain fibres are stimulated and a powerful impulse shoots up the sensory nerve into the posterior grey matter of the spinal cord; the impulse is immediately relayed to cells in the anterior horn and these directly initiate impulses in the motor nerves which will result in accurate withdrawal from the stimulus. Milliseconds *later* pain is appreciated in consciousness (Figure 1). This withdrawal mechanism is the fastest reflex in the body, and it is *prepotent*; in other words it takes precedence over any other reflex, however caused.

The whole question of the purpose of these mechanisms will be dealt with in the next part, but we might note here a definition of pain by the neurologist Sir Charles Sherrington – 'the psychical adjunct of an imperative protective reflex.' (This definition covers only a fraction of the spectrum of pain.) The withdrawal reflex can be overcome or inhibited by an effort of will in certain circumstances. A sudden severe unexpected harmful stimulus to the body surface such as a stab or a burn will almost invariably cause reflex withdrawal (if such movement is possible) but if the stimulus is not too severe, and if he knows it is coming, a man can train himself not to react to it, in other words he can modify his natural reflex by a conscious process which can exceptionally be carried to extremes. This is apparently accomplished by a stream of impulses travelling down from the higher centres and interrupting the normal circuit at one of the relay points.[1]

The Varieties of Surface Pain

The animal's surface constitutes its immediate contact with its environment, being exposed to every kind of possible harm. So on the surface pain can be accurately localized and the withdrawal reflex is immediate and dependable. As we recede from the surface localization becomes steadily less accurate, though this does not mean that deep pain is less severe; it may be intense. Also the skin is able to differentiate between many different kinds of noxious stimuli (though not all kinds) conveying the appropriate information into consciousness, whereas deeper structures may only be sensitive to special stimuli and no automatic withdrawal mechanism is provided.

In the skin we are able to distinguish between pricking, cutting, tearing, crushing and burning pains. In addition we can estimate their severity to some extent, and localize the point of injury very

[1] Ronald Melzack, in *Scientific American*, February, 1961.

accurately. It must be admitted that the differentiation between cutting, burning and so on may depend very largely on the simultaneous stimulation of other special sensory nerve endings; also on the knowledge, by sight or sound or even smell, that the pain is going to be caused by (for instance) a bite, or a red-hot iron or a knife. A man blindfolded and touched briefly on the skin with a red-hot needle may accurately localize a severe pain but be quite unable to say whether it was caused by a hot or a very cold object or by a stab or a cut. Some physiologists think that the pain of a burn is produced by the simultaneous stimulation of nerve endings sensitive to *warmth* and those conveying pain; and similarly with other typical pains.

The severity of the pain is only an extremely rough indication of the degree of injury, many other factors being involved. During World War II, Henry K. Beecher of the Harvard Medical School personally observed the behaviour of soldiers severely wounded in battle.[1] He found that the severity of the wound had very little relation to the amount of pain apparently produced, and in some extremely severe injuries the main emotional response was thankfulness at escaping alive from the battlefield, pain being declared to be minimal or absent. By contrast electric shocks may be acutely painful, but produce practically no physical injury.

Skin Sensitivity

On the whole the front of the body is more sensitive to pain than the back, the finger tips and the lips particularly so. The lobe of the ear is fairly insensitive and can be pierced with little pain, but a slight jab with the same needle under a nail is excruciating. Many other examples could be given but the matter is one of common experience. Less obvious perhaps is the variation in any one situation under different conditions. Sensitiveness can be reduced markedly by inattention, cold, drugs and certain diseases, notably those affecting the nervous system; it is increased by concentration on the part, by emotional factors and by local inflammation however caused.

[1] *Pain, an International Symposium*, ed. R. S. Knighton and P. Dumke.

These are only examples; the subject of threshold is dealt with in more detail later.

Interruption of the Pathway

If the sensory nerve pathway is interrupted at any point on its way to consciousness the experience of pain will be diminished or lost. We have just seen one example – the application of cocaine to the nerve endings. Cutting the sensory nerves or the tracts in the spinal cord will have the same effect; so will destruction of certain areas in the brain, but owing to the wide connections between these areas the effects are not wholly predictable. Also even if the impulses reach the brain they may be prevented from entering consciousness by various drugs and by subtle psychological processes (see Part IV).

A good deal of our knowledge about pain pathways comes from studying the results of such interruptions by disease and injury, and by the deliberate section of nerves. The psychological aspects present far greater problems, mostly unsolved, yet these are of the utmost importance in our attempts to understand pain.

The Autonomic Nervous System

A special sub-division of the nervous system known as the Autonomic System carries the responsibility for control of *involuntary muscle*. This kind of muscle, which is not under conscious control, is found in the hollow viscera (stomach, intestine, bladder, uterus and others) as well as in the heart and blood vessels, in the lungs and in many glands. In some cases it provides a double innervation known as *sympathetic* and *para-sympathetic*, usually having opposite effects such as contraction and relaxation; the activity of some organs is the result of a very accurate balance between the two sets of fibres. To complicate matters still further, both sympathetic and para-sympathetic nerves may carry sensory fibres as well as motor ones and these are capable of conveying special kinds of pain. Many painful conditions result from impulses originating in both the cerebrospinal and the Autonomic systems. This fact may account for some of the peculiarities of 'referred pain', which we shall encounter again a little later. For instance, sympathetic pain fibres from part of the stomach enter the spinal cord at the level of the fifth cervical nerve roots in the neck, and this segment of the cord also receives ordinary pain nerves from an area of skin just below the sternum (breast-bone). In certain circumstances pain of gastric origin is felt in this area of skin.

PAIN BELOW THE SURFACE

If the appropriate stimulus is applied pain can be elicited in most tissues and organs; yet many of these are completely insensitive to damage that would cause intense pain in the skin.

The subcutaneous tissues are specially sensitive to stretching and to chemical irritants – a fact amply proved by the effect of certain injections.

Muscle reacts to the accumulation of substances normally removed by the circulating blood. If a muscle is exercised to such a degree that the production of waste exceeds the capacity of the circulation to remove it, severe pain develops. Experimentally this is easily demonstrated by exercising a limb with a tourniquet on it; the pain is relieved by removing the tourniquet. Ordinary skeletal muscle is also sensitive to crushing and to various chemical substances injected into it such as Penicillin. The type of muscle found elsewhere in the body (involuntary muscle) is dealt with under visceral pain (page 28). Intense spasm in any muscle causes severe pain, including the muscle in the walls of arteries.

Bone itself is not so pain-sensitive as is commonly supposed, the loose spongy kind of bone being much more so than compact dense bone; the membrane covering bone (periosteum) is acutely sensitive to pain. The special bone of teeth is quite insensitive to cutting and drilling until the dentine and the pulp are involved, and these can cause very acute pain when insulted, as we all know. These structures are also exquisitely sensitive to temperature, to sugar (hot sweet tea!) and curiously (and uniquely) to tiny electric currents such as those generated between a metal dental filling and some other metal like a knife blade or a key. Severe toothache is caused when the dentine or pulp are exposed by decay. This dentine is one comparatively superficial tissue in the body (others are the ear-drum and the conjunctiva covering the front of the eye) which convey no sensation other than pain; this is characteristic of all deep tissues, and of almost the entire gastro-intestinal tract. Exceptions are the sensations of heat and cold detected by the oesophagus (gullet) and by the lower part of the rectum, and the deep sensations associated with the sexual reflexes.

Joints are surrounded by ligaments which are sensitive to stretching (sprain). The smooth articular *cartilage* of joints can be cut or burned without pain, but the delicate membranes secreting the lubricating fluid (synovial membranes) causes severe pain when quite gently stimulated mechanically or with chemicals.

Nerve tissue is of special interest as a source of pain. The brain itself is not sensitive to burning or cutting although its blood vessels and its coverings (meninges) can be very painful. In the wild it is unnecessary for the brain to be sensitive as damage is nearly always fatal; the fact that neuro-surgeons are able to do something about it is not relevant in this particular connection. Sensory nerves become very tender when they are inflamed (Neuritis). We have already seen that interruption of a pain pathway anywhere between the nerve ending and consciousness will lead to diminution or absence of pain in the part concerned. Similarly, a stimulus applied at any point in the pathway may lead to a sensation of pain, and this pain is felt in the part of the body from which the nerve comes. This stimulus may arise from neuritis, various kinds of neuralgia, diseases such as herpes and, of course, from a mechanical injury.

A curious example of this type of phenomenon from the realm of surgery is known as the '*phantom limb*', first described by the surgeon Ambroise Paré in 1552. In the course of an operation for amputation of a leg at mid-thigh, for instance, all the different tissues have to be divided — skin, fat, membranes, muscles, blood vessels, bone and nerves. Now nearly all the nerves of the lower limb are gathered together in the thigh to form the *sciatic nerve*, the largest nerve in the body, about half an inch thick. When this has been cut impulses continue to pass up its fibres from irritation of the severed ends, and the brain and mind interpret these as stimuli from the various nerve endings (Figure 5). It therefore appears to the patient that he still has his leg, and since all sensory fibres are represented in the sciatic nerve he feels his leg orientated in space and related to touch, temperature, position and pain, so a few amputees (fortunately very few) feel acute pain in a limb that no longer exists, and this may last for twenty-five years or even longer. After a time this kind of sensation may become fixed centrally and when this happens even section of the sensory pathways by operation will fail to abolish the pain (see Part IV). This unfortunate condition has of course been the subject of psychiatric study, and in some circles the patient's suffering has been ascribed to 'mourning' for the lost limb.

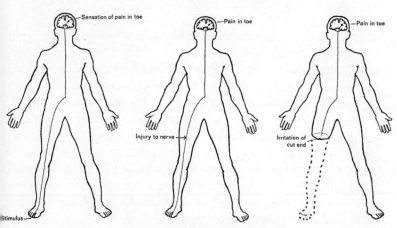

Fig. 5. The Phantom Limb

Perhaps even more distressing (who can tell?) is severe pain felt in a limb or other part that is completely normal, because of interference with the sensory nerve pathway at a higher level. An example is the agonising pain in one side of the face and head due to disease of the fifth cranial (trigeminal) nerve, and known as Trigeminal Neuralgia or *tic douloureux*. Here the pain may start spontaneously or it may be precipitated by the slightest stimulation of the skin — even by a draught of cold air. The wretched sufferer dares not shave or wash for fear of an attack and this produces secondary skin changes that themselves can act as the trigger. Surgery provides the only relief (Part IV).

Another example is the familiar 'slipped disc' causing pain in the leg. In this case compression takes place within the vertebral column itself by the escape of the jelly-like 'ball-bearings' between the individual vertebra. If this happens (as it usually does) in the lower part of the back the main sensory pathways affected are those conveyed from the leg in the sciatic nerve and the result is the pain down the back of the leg known as *sciatica*. There are a great many other possible causes of sciatica, and correct diagnosis is very important.

Visceral Pain

This means pain arising in the different organs of the body, as well as in some other tissues. There are certain curious features about the distribution of such pain that are sometimes hard to explain, but the characteristic features have been extensively studied and are of the utmost value in the diagnosis of disease; this aspect will be examined in more detail in Part II. Here we are more concerned with the origins of these pains, with their relative sensitiveness and with the type of pain produced.

The heart and its enclosing membrane (pericardium) are insensitive to direct injury, but like any other muscular organ the heart reacts with pain to being deprived of its blood supply. Heart muscle is supplied with its own blood vessels known as the *coronary arteries*. If these are narrowed or blocked by disease the muscle suffers because it cannot stop to rest; waste products build up and pain is felt. Complete blockage of all the coronary arteries results in death.

Pain of this kind is rarely felt over the heart itself, but is *referred* to sites like the back, the inner side of the left arm and the jaws. The reason for this is thought to be that the Autonomic sensory nerve fibres from the heart enter the spinal cord at the same levels as do ordinary sensory fibres from these varied situations, and incoming impulses are radiated to adjacent nerve cells; one of the curiosities of medicine is pain of this kind felt in an arm that in fact no longer exists, having been amputated some years previously. Pain felt over the heart itself can have a variety of causes, most of them more frightening than serious; the term 'angina pectoris' is usually applied to severe intermittent pain of cardiac origin but not necessarily due to actual coronary artery disease. Some cases seem to be caused by spasm of these arteries, and the pain can be relieved by special relaxing drugs.

Blood vessels (like most tissues) are sensitive to stretching, crushing, to electrical stimuli, to the insertion of needles and to spasm of their intrinsic muscle. Since nearly all tissues contain arteries suitable stimuli can give rise to pain in them. They convey no sensation apart from pain.

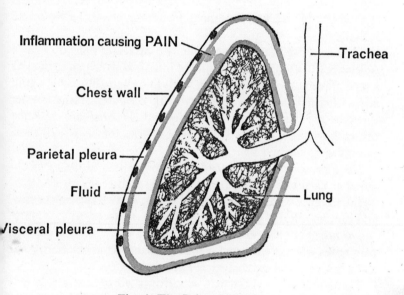

Fig. 6. The Pain of Pleurisy

Lung tissue itself is quite insensitive, so is the membrane that encloses it (the visceral pleura); a second layer of pleura continuous with the first (the parietal pleura) lines the inside of the chest wall, an arrangement that permits the lung to move freely because there is normally a thin film of slippery fluid between the two layers (Figure 6). The parietal pleura is acutely sensitive to injury or infection; if it gets roughened the friction with lung movements causes the pain known as pleurisy, which is particularly vivid when a deep breath is attempted.

Most parts of the *intestine*, from the stomach to the upper part of the rectum, enjoy a considerable degree of mobility, and this is facilitated by an arrangement rather similar to the two layers of pleura. Both the intestine itself and the inside of the abdominal cavity are lined with the thin glossy moist *peritoneum*. An exposed loop of normal bowel, covered with peritoneum, is completely insensitive to cutting, burning or crushing. However, the same peritoneum is sensitive to stretching, as in a very distended bowel. The peritoneal lining of the abdominal wall is sensitive to mechanical and chemical stimuli, and the pain of *peritonitis* is due to its chemical stimulation by released intestinal matter or blood, or by severe infection.

The bowel itself can produce pain by contracting violently against resistance (for example in any kind of intestinal obstruction) causing a type of pain called '*colic*', which tends to be periodic. Colicky pain arises when any hollow muscular structure contracts violently; other examples are the pain from gallstones and kidney stones, and that resulting from the sudden blockage of arteries (embolus); all these can cause agonizing pain.

The liver, kidneys, spleen and pancreas are insensitive to mechanical or chemical stimuli; pain arising from these organs is caused by interference with their own blood vessels or with adjacent organs, and is often referred to various parts of the surface.

The uterus (womb) can be cut and burnt without any sensation; pain arises when it contracts against resistance as in childbirth, but there is a powerful psychological element here.

The testicle is the most pain-sensitive of all organs, a fact well known to those concerned with the infliction of pain. This particular pain shares with some others the property of being 'sickening' in character.

CHARACTERISTICS OF THE PAIN SENSE

With a gradually increasing superficial stimulus the nerves of pain start transmission just *before* actual tissue damage starts. A homely example of this is lying in a bath and adding water from the hot tap, with of course some rather primitive stirring activity, so that the heat increases slowly until it reaches that of 'a nice hot bath'; a few degrees above this and it begins to hurt. The pain threshold may vary between individuals but if they are healthy it is nearly always below the point at which actual skin damage occurs. This is characteristic of all superficial pain, however caused, though certain kinds of skin damage such as frostbite and sunburn can occur without any pain at the time of applying the stimulus. The pain may be out of all proportion to the triviality of the disease process, as in some kinds of neuralgia; on the other hand there may be little or no pain from very extensive wounds.

The Effects of Disease

Any tissue that is pain-sensitive when normal becomes very much more so (hyperalgesia) when *inflamed*, and this may also cause certain tissues normally insensitive to become painful. A common result of inflammation is pulsation of the pain (throbbing) with each heart beat, due to the increased tension in the arteries and cells in the tissues. An inflamed finger is exquisitely tender; it throbs, and the pain is eased slightly by raising the hand above the level of the heart so reducing the pressure in the blood vessels. The delicate membranes enclosing the brain (the meninges) are mainly insensitive but give rise to severe pain with certain types of inflammation (meningitis). Most *growths* are themselves quite insensitive, being indeed devoid of nerves; they may cause pain by invasion of, or pressure upon, sensitive structures such as bone, periosteum, or nerves themselves. Some diseases and growths have the reverse effect; by destroying nerve tissue they cause absence of pain or complete numbness. This is specially characteristic of various diseases affecting the spinal cord. On the other hand a rare condition affecting the thalamus itself results in gross exaggeration of all pain sensations however caused, so that for instance a minor prick with a needle in the back of the hand causes agonising pain. The place of disease will be dealt with in more detail in various references to the medical aspects of pain.

The Bodily Response to Severe Pain

We shall see later that the total response of a human being to bad pain depends very much on his emotional attitude towards it — the usual immediate emotional reaction is in fact astonishment that it can be so bad; this is something that cannot be imagined beforehand, and incidentally is very difficult to remember later. Just now we are more concerned with the more automatic physiological responses, and these again are varied according to the site and cause of the pain. However, if a comparatively simple example is taken the response can be predicted with some accuracy.

Severe superficial pain is produced when heat is applied to the skin, perhaps in the form of a burn by hot iron. The immediate withdrawal reflex has already been mentioned. Pain is then consciously appreciated, and vocal expression is commonly given by screaming or cursing or both. If the pain continues and escape is impossible struggling efforts are made and these may be accompanied by moaning, weeping and by various facial contortions; there is an initial rise of blood pressure, the pupils dilate, the victim becomes pale and sweats profusely, his breathing changes to a rapid gasping kind, his pulse rate is increased, and then his blood pressure falls; if it falls far enough he may lose consciousness, now being in a state of 'shock'. All these responses, except perhaps cursing, can be observed in the higher animals (especially in the mammalian vertebrates) and while we cannot extrapolate to the extent of crediting them with our own emotional reactions it must be quite obvious that they feel pain. There are some specious philosophical arguments that they do not, and these are mainly supported (though not understood) by the devotees of certain sports involving animals. The controversy regarding blood sports should not include arguments about whether they cause pain or not — they do.

The further physical effects of pain depend mainly on the extent to which it inhibits normal functions such as sleeping, feeding and moving about; both these and the immediate responses can be greatly enhanced or minimized by emotional factors such as fear, anger, resentment, devotion, repentance and ecstasy. There are also wide variations in individual pain thresholds, but responses tend to be more uniform at extremes.

The Subjective Varieties of Pain

Superficial pain is usually described in terms of the causative agent, for instance as stabbing, cutting, or burning. As we have seen these varieties are not entirely separated anatomically and may be deduced through other simultaneous sensation. Deeper pains may be similarly described but present additional types that do not occur in the skin; thus we experience cramp-like muscular pains, the frightening pain of a coronary attack, and the violent wrenching pain of renal colic. Headache, earache and toothache are unique pains with every degree of intensity. Deeper still pain may be diffuse and undefinable, occupying (for instance) the whole of the abdomen, with many possible causes. The pain may be intermittent or continuous; sharp or aching; necessary or apparently pointless; with an end in view, or hopeless.

THRESHOLD AND CAPACITY

It is a matter of common experience that some people are 'soft' and others 'tough', certainly so far as the middle degrees of pain are concerned; this is susceptible to actual measurement scientifically and many studies have been made. The general lines of such experiments are to use standard graded stimuli such as hot test tubes, electric currents, the open-blisters technique referred to on pp. 17 and 18, and the tourniquet method for muscular pain. These stimuli are applied to volunteers with increasing severity until they are declared to be painful or intolerable. Of course under these conditions such psychic potentiators such as fear, despair and distress are absent; in fact there is a certain compulsion to see how much one can actually stand.

Experimental work of this kind and clinical observations in practice all confirm the common impression of great variation, particularly regarding the ability to stand moderately severe pain. At very low levels pain tends to begin at a point just below that at which damage occurs and differences are not great except where local changes would limit damage anyway, as in the horny hands of manual labourers. But at moderately severe levels individuals differ very markedly in their resistance, and this has often been commented on, perhaps sometimes with a tendency to bias. 'There is little doubt that in the lower classes the sensation of pain is felt in a much less degree than in those of a highly intellectual and nervous temperament.'[1] One extensive survey showed abnormally high tolerance in American Indians, prize-fighters and Negroes, and another in Russian peasants. The condition does seem to be related to some extent with low intelligence-quotients, but no general conclusions can be drawn about this.

Of course it is not possible to measure the amount of pain a man actually feels, only the strength of the stimulus applied and his physiological reactions, such as pulse rate, blood pressure and sweating. Over many years, observation of patients after surgical operations leads to the conclusion that some people simply do not react to conditions that cause intense pain in others – a circumstance that makes the evaluation of analgesics very difficult in anything but very extended trials (page 134, Part IV). This is particularly evident in fairly standardized procedures such as most hernia operations and straightforward 'interval' removal of the appendix. Some people suffer quite a lot, can't sleep, and need a powerful analgesic drug by injection. Others simply declare that they have no pain, and sleep like a log without drugs of any kind. One regularly encounters individuals who seem to have little or no pain after really extensive and mutilating procedures like amputations or radical mastectomy (complete removal of the breast), and I would further say that it is almost impossible to predict their reactions beforehand. Moreover the effect is seen in men and women of all ages, and even in quite young children.

Attention and Attitude

You will sometimes hear it said that pain is a purely mental phenomenon, therefore it only exists in people's minds, and so it has no 'real' existence. This argument carries little weight with the patient suffering from renal colic or a man being tortured.

[1] *Anomalies and Curiosities of Medicine*, G. M. Gould and W. L. Pyle (1897).

All forms of sensation ultimately reach consciousness and are translated into various kinds of experience; from these we arrive at conclusions about what is happening around us and within our bodies. Pain is perhaps the most subjective of all sensations — we do not project it outside ourselves in the way we do with sight, sounds and feelings, and even smells. The moment pain occurs it becomes intensely personal, and although it may result from external physical events it is not felt to exist at all outside the body. This of course tends to focus attention on the hurt part and so to increase awareness, and it is very much more difficult to shut it out in the way some other sensations can be manipulated. We can shut our eyes, or look somewhere else; sound is more diffuse, but one can concentrate on the single component in a mass of sounds, with practice almost exclusively; taste and smell can be analysed to an extent that the untrained find astonishing. But severe pain is insistent, crude and utterly dominant, claiming all the attention available, and clamouring for action.

The more attention is devoted to any sensation the more acutely it is perceived, and *vice versa*. Pain is no exception — the less attention you pay to it the less you feel it; but the extreme difficulty is to divert attention from such an intense experience — the very effort to do so has exactly the reverse effect. Pain such as toothache is worst when there are no diversions of any kind, as in the quiet stillness of the night: one may get up, wander around the house, try to read or do some work, and eventually sheer weariness may take precedence; if sleep comes, pain ceases to exist.

A man working on some project of extreme interest can sustain cuts and bruises without feeling them at all. He finds them later, having been completely unaware of the stimulus. Exactly the same injuries produced deliberately would hurt considerably. In unusual circumstances quite severe injuries can occur without pain; this complete diversion of attention can be induced in a fully conscious subject by hypnosis. In the ordinary way however we have astonishingly little control over our own minds — small pains and nagging worries tend to occupy high degrees of attention in spite of (or because of) all our efforts, and we envy the rare individuals who are to some extent able to 'switch off'. Can this ability be acquired by training? Apparently it can, but only with enormous effort, or by hypnosis. The rigid mental disciplines imposed by certain varieties of Yoga, and by the esoteric practices of some religions, may enable the practitioner to achieve an extraordinary degree of concentration; and this implies the complete exclusion of things outside the object of concentration, perhaps even extending to severe pain. The further claims that such practices lead (or *may* lead, with grace) to spiritual enlightenment are completely unknowable except to those who have actually experienced them, though it is said that they can be simulated by drugs of the Lysergic acid type.

A man may tolerate quite severe pain if he knows it has an object, as in treatment, or if it is purely experimental and will be instantly withdrawn if he says the word. The woman in labour may stand severe pain, especially if the baby is a wanted one, even more so if she has been trained to relax and accept it (page 145).

Indifference to pain can certainly be acquired by constant practice, and if this is the sole object of one's existence can be carried to extremes, as in the case of some fakirs. Similar exhibitions are sometimes seen in side-shows at fairs,[1] and in minor degrees the phenomenon is commonplace. Even quite small children can be trained to give themselves injections, of insulin for example, and eventually seem to be unaware of any pain when the needle enters the skin.

People who meet pain with philosophical acceptance bear it better than those who resent and fear it. Those sustained by profound faith are better equipped than those without such anchors — the faith can be almost anything, including themselves; but it must be the kind that moves mountains, that is 'more aggressive than evidence' (Edwin G. Boring) — not the kind defined by the schoolboy as 'believing what you know to be untrue'.

The converse is far easier and commoner; increase of pain by psychic potentiation. In the days of the Inquisition the Question began by taking the victim to the torture-chamber and exhibiting in detail the various instruments that could be used — the rack, pulleys, the fire and so on. This often succeeded without further ado, but if it did not the effect of the subsequent proceedings was greatly enhanced by anticipation and fear. (The Gestapo employed precisely similar techniques.)

[1] *Memoirs of a Sword Swallower*, Dan Mannix.

PSYCHOGENIC PAIN

Before leaving this section on the pathways of pain we must refer
to the kind that arises near the end of the path – pain that finds origin
in the devious labyrinths of the mind.

There is a tendency to label all pain for which no physical basis
can be found as psychogenic, sometimes a convenient method of
hiding ignorance. There can be a great variety of reasons for a complaint of pain, ranging from an inoperable cancer to sheer malingering: a large remainder includes psychic factors in different degrees,
and there are probably three main categories.

1. Almost everyone at times gets fleeting transient pains in
different parts of the body – minor headaches, slight indigestion,
little stabs in the joints, aching muscles after unaccustomed exercise,
and so on. The chronic worrier's mind seizes on these trivia and
magnifies them into possible major disease. He cannot help doing
this and indeed very often knows about his weakness, but this
knowledge does not make his pain any less. You will see that one
cannot say his pain is not real – it is, and he needs help.

2. The effect of mental tension is often to cause muscular tension, with a predilection for certain groups of muscles. Among these
are the occipito-frontalis muscles of the scalp, causing not only a
wrinkled brow but a special type of headache. There seems no
doubt that pain in the back, the neck, the abdomen and probably
other parts can be so caused, and even sometimes relieved by
conscious relaxation.

These two categories are currently described as *psychosomatic*
conditions.

3. True psychogenic pain, in which the coded pain-pattern is
impressed on consciousness from the vast nebulous world of the
unconscious, is probably uncommon. Its origins may lie in half-
formulated resentment against real or imagined wrongs, or perhaps
in a form of self-punishment, an attempt to atone for long forgotten sins. The process by which repressed material leads to anxiety
and thence to functional disorders, including pain, is technically
known as a *conversion reaction*. After a time this process can lead to
secondary physical effects, and the picture becomes very complicated.

The extent to which actual organic disease can be caused by mental processes is not well understood, and there are differences of opinion about this. There seems little doubt that duodenal ulcers (for instance) and chronic ulceration in the lower bowel can follow the continuous local spasm induced by psychic tensions. How far this process is reversible is still more controversial, but it would appear logical that the relief of tension and hence of intestinal spasm could provide suitable conditions for the natural cure of some of these diseases. At least one faith-healer makes a speciality of gastric ulcers, claiming radiological proof of success. For a number of reasons the technique is not usable by orthodox practitioners.

It can readily be appreciated that these are not clear-cut categories and may co-exist in any combination, making diagnosis and treatment difficult. In regard to pain with a true psychogenic origin one wonders if it is not a real necessity to some of these patients, and if efforts to eradicate it may occasionally do more harm than good.

There is no clear-cut distinction between true psychogenic pain and malingering (conscious deception) — cases often have components of both. So far as 'imaginary' pain is concerned some people are very surprised at the result of a simple psychological experiment, which consists in sitting quietly with the eyes shut and concentrating the entire attention on some part of the body, perhaps the right thumb, imagining it to be swollen and inflamed and throbbing with pain. After a few minutes one often begins to feel actual pain in the part, and with practice it can become quite severe. A very curious feature of this situation is that the self-induced pain does not disappear the moment concentration ceases, but lasts for several minutes, or occasionally much longer.

It begins to look as if pain is a vastly complex phenomenon occupying a large part of our intricate nervous system. Surely there is some purpose in all this? The withdrawal reflex clearly has a useful function, but it by-passes consciousness. Why then do we feel pain?

PART TWO

THE PURPOSE AND ACCEPTABLE USES OF PAIN

THE PURPOSE

THE WORD PURPOSE is used here with the ordinary meaning that everyone understands, entirely free from philosophical connotations. There is no sense in straining to avoid a good word just because a few people might draw unjustified conclusions of a teleological nature from it.

Pain is so universal and powerful an experience that man has always felt the need to explain its existence. Perhaps the earliest of all rationalizations was that pain is the punishment for Sin, an opinion that dies hard. The extreme opposite – also a religious view – is that pain does not really exist at all, we simply imagine it does. This is a particularly interesting opinion, especially when considered in relation to the many psychological aspects of pain, and we shall see that pain can indeed be abolished by purely mental processes in certain circumstances.

The narrowest scientific thinking places pain as a protective reflex mechanism essential for survival, and while this may not be the whole story it has the backing of cold reason, so we might begin by examining the evolution of pain as a biological necessity for higher animals, originating in a simple escape from harmful stimuli by the most primitive creature deserving the term 'animal'.

The *Amoeba*, which some of us remember with affection under microscopes at school, is composed of a single cell – a minute blob of protoplasm equipped with a nucleus and other curious structures; it lives in pond water and possesses all the basic functions we associate with living animals—moving, feeding, excreting and reproducing. It accomplishes these by changes in its shape.

The amoeba (Figure 7, page 42) feeds by a kind of 3D pincer movement, flowing round a fragment of organic material and then digesting it. Any undigested residue is extruded by a similar process in reverse. It follows that the creature is equipped with some

41

mechanism for distinguishing food particles from useless or harmful stimuli, and in fact it retreats from the latter by changing its shape and flowing away. We can study this process by prodding the amoeba with extremely fine glass points made by the familiar method of pulling out heated glass rods into filaments. The amoeba recoils from such an attack and flows away.

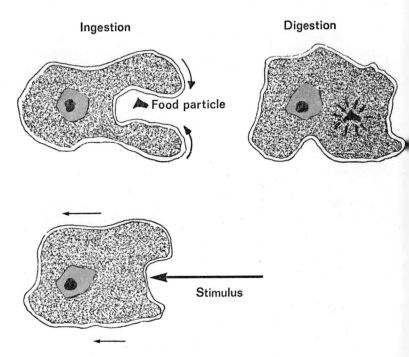

Fig. 7. The Amoeba

Here we have a primitive withdrawal mechanism; it is not a true *reflex*—the amoeba has no nerves; and it would be pushing anthropomorphism to a ridiculous extent to say that it was 'cruel'—the creature cannot feel pain, for it has no nervous system and no brain. This withdrawal from noxious agents is fundamental in the animal kingdom and it is obviously advantageous, in that any creature not so equipped will succumb to predators without the hope of escape.

Multi-cellular Creatures

All higher creatures have a great many cells, and as they become more complex different groups of cells become specialized for various functions. Clearly some form of co-ordination must exist between these groups and the cells composing them so that the animal can act as a whole. Initially in animals with only a few cells, this seems to take place by exchange of information directly between adjacent cells, and recent work suggests that this is done by the actual passage of large molecules between them. Eventually (in animals) this co-ordinating factor becomes the special respon-sibility of the *nervous system* — in close co-operation with a chemical system distributed by the blood stream. On the whole the chemical system lacks the immediacy of the nervous system though both are vital. An animal must be equipped with the means of escape from harm, and those that lack this would not last long in the struggle for existence. At first the simple withdrawal reflex would be enough, but the creature that kept barging into harmful objects, even if it could withdraw quickly, would soon suffer damage and a means must exist whereby it learns from experience. This mechanism exists in quite lowly creatures. An octopus 'likes' small crabs to eat and it 'dislikes' electric shocks. It will make several attacks on crabs in spite of being given a shock every time, but eventually it does learn; associating 'crab' with 'shock' it will remain curled up in a corner of its tank and refuse to attack the proffered crab.[1]

I have used several words in this very condensed account of a significant experiment that imply human thought processes and emotions, and this is certainly not a valid interpretation; one word I have not used is 'pain', though one can surely see the beginnings of the pain system at this level.

We can go a stage further, performing a similar experiment with a vastly more highly developed animal, a dog. Initially the reaction appears the same: the dog is offered food but cannot reach it without getting an electric shock which it feels as a mildly painful sensation and dislikes. Later it tries again but caution is evident very soon, and the food is refused after a few tries. But now persist until the animal is really hungry; it will force itself to sustain the shock in

[1] J. Z. Young, *Doubt and Certainty in Science*, Reith Lectures, 1950.

order to get the food. Still more remarkable is that eventually the dog will appear to take the shock as a matter of course, apparently feeling negligible discomfort, so long as it is associated with a satisfactory meal, and it will even give itself a shock if this is necessary to obtain food. Pavlov went considerably further than this and conditioned dogs to accept burns as the price of a meal, eventually apparently without undue discomfort.

Let us now return to the child who touches the fire. We saw how sensory impulses from the burnt finger travelled to the spinal cord, were short-circuited there and gave rise to motor impulses resulting in withdrawal; a fraction of a second later the impulse enters consciousness and is appreciated as pain accurately located in that finger. The child now possesses a mass of information about the fire and its effects; extrapolation will enable it to *recognize* fire again, by sight and by the remote cutaneous appreciation of heat rays; the association with *pain* shows that direct contact with fire is to be avoided, so in future anything obviously hot is approached with caution—and so, in a similar way, is anything else that experience identifies as a cause of pain and therefore of potential harm. This is particularly important in cases where the conscious part may be the only association, as in the case of *sunburn* where the pain develops some hours after the harmful stimulus. It does not protect the victim on the first occasion, but he learns by bitter experience not to repeat it. This *conscious* learning by experience is obviously a great advance on the more primitive method, and creatures endowed with it will climb the evolutionary scale more rapidly than the rest. The more one thinks about it the more one realizes that a necessary part of this process is the sensation we know as pain, something very unpleasant, something we dislike and try to avoid.

There are several other examples of this particular aspect in relation to the function of pain in our lives.

Perhaps the most sensitive surface we present to the outside world is that of the eye, the conjunctiva. It literally weeps at the smallest insult. It is practically the shortest distance from the brain and the blink reflex in response to the slightest threat is the fastest in the body. We learn by the experience of pain to avoid exposing this delicate organ to any abnormal stimulus. The automatic response is the production of tears to dilute the irritation, but weeping is one of the responses to any kind of pain, for reasons not easy to analyse.

Overstrain

Consider once again the proposition that pain, however caused, is an indication of actual or potential harm to the body. During the course of work and play we subject the structures of our bodies to many kinds of violence: the labourer at his work, the stoker, the man digging in his garden, the athlete pole-vaulting. In each case the surface of the body, the muscles and the structures composing joints are frequently subjected to violence, yet actual injury is comparatively rare, unless something unforeseen happens, because *pain* in the structures concerned warns the individual that the point of danger is being reached. Notice here the operation of a principle known in engineering as 'feed-back'. The man is straining to move a stiff lever; sensory impulses from the skin of his hands and from many parts of his body pass up hundreds of nerves, and the co-ordinated information is 'processed' by millions of cells in the brain; the result is a series of motor impulses operating precisely those muscles that will apply efficient power to the lever; probably orientations and tensions in the entire body are involved. It is easy to see that in a total effort of this kind one muscle might easily be over-strained with consequent damage, but each and every part involved sends back streams of messages as to its particular state and these influence the distribution of effort. Normally such a balance is unconscious, but misapplication of effort due to inexperience (or some reaction by the object) may over-strain one part; the development of pain impulses not only guards the part at once but warns against the future application of similar efforts.

Countless examples could be given of this function of *warning* about potential damage, plus *learning* by experience to avoid similar contingencies, but this concept of pain is a rather obvious one. Protection in this way is vitally necessary to our delicate organism, and indeed without it we could certainly not exist at all, for we would not have survived the hazards of evolution to our present state. However, this is not by any means the whole story of pain, and we must now try to search for the more subtle aspects.

Man and his Environment

Man has developed to a fantastic degree the ability to survive and function in adverse conditions. I am not comparing him with *seeds* that withstand drying and freezing for years[1] and *spores* that survive boiling – these are not functioning creatures. Man has proved his ability to live and work in polar cold, in tropical heat, in the depths of the sea and in the vacuum of space. No animal can approach this performance unless aided by man, cosseted in his clothes, enclosed in his vehicles, warmed or cooled by his crafty apparatus.

Completely unaided, Man is a weak and pitiful creature; one writer has compared him with 'an unborn ape'. All the clothing and the protection are necessary because he is so vulnerable, so highly differentiated from his environment; like any other animal his life is a constant struggle 'to prevent his organization being disrupted by damage and disease' (J. Z. Young), and one of the vital mechanisms is that of pain.

The 'organization' referred to by Professor Young is the animal's state of biological equilibrium with its environment. In the case of man, this is very intricate indeed; the happy comfortable man must be satisfied nutritionally and sexually – the ambient temperature and the water balance must be right – gravitational and postural effects must impose no strain – light must not be too bright nor noise too loud – his entire organization must be functioning correctly and he must be free from disease – and finally he must be free from psychological disturbances. In other words there must be no actual or anticipated or imagined harm. If there is, disturbing messages flow into the brain; these lead, in minor degrees, to discomfort – in major degrees, to pain.

---

[1] Seeds of the Arctic Lupin, frozen for at least 10,000 years, have germinated and actually produced flowers under laboratory conditions in Canada. (*New Scientist*, October 19th, 1967.)

Injury and Disease

Fast and efficient as it is, the protective reflex mechanism is not infallible. From time to time various parts of the body suffer damage by direct injury or by the manifold forms of disease; many of these insults lead to pain, and most of these pains are strongly resented by human recipients. Let us see how far the experience of pain from such sources can be justified on biological grounds.

The body has very remarkable powers of self-repair: the healing of superficial wounds is taken for granted and can be observed by everyone; cracks in bones, fractured skulls, broken ribs, torn ligaments, some damaged organs – all are capable of healing in time. We recover from the onslaught of many diseases without any medical aid: pneumonia, heart disease, malaria, boils – each leaves its mark, but recovery of the organism as a whole is *possible*, given a chance; and the biggest chance that unaided nature can be given is rest.

The Importance of Rest

One of the most significant medical text books ever published was *Rest and Pain*, based on a series of lectures given by John Hilton to the Royal College of Surgeons in 1862. In those days there were no specific remedies for disease in the sense that antibiotics are today, but a great number of spurious, harmful and barbarous methods of treatment were in constant use. Hilton's creed was that if the affected part was placed at rest, nature would heal it if that were possible, and the great indicator for rest was pain. In broad outline this may seem obvious but, the healing processes themselves are very intricate. Let us consider some examples of this mechanism.

A sudden twist inwards of the foot may result in tearing the powerful ligaments on the outer side, the so-called *sprained ankle*. Intense pain occurs, exaggerated by the slightest attempt to repeat the movement; walking is almost impossible, and a position of comparative ease is found with the foot turned slightly outwards and the leg elevated. In this position the injured parts are brought together and swelling is minimized, the torn ligaments re-form, at first weakly and later to full strength. If the destructive force were repeated at this stage the healing processes would be violently disturbed, but such movements are normally prevented by sheer pain. In about two weeks tentative efforts at use are possible and as the repair becomes stronger further liberties can be taken, until at last all ordinary movements are painless and the ligaments have soundly healed.

Notice that use or strapping or splints or plaster in such a condition is merely an aid to rest. The original injury to a joint may be very painful, but attempts to move it a few days later are agonizing; few victims could withstand a second session on the rack.

The pain of a *coronary thrombosis* is of a peculiarly alarming character, leading usually to breathlessness and immediate cessation of all effort. Part of the heart muscle is deprived of its blood supply and the slightest increase in its work leads to further local accumulations of waste products. Pain is usually felt in the arm or back or jaws or abdomen—rarely, if ever, over the heart itself. The victim's only chance of recovery is to keep the cardiac output down to the absolute minimum, and initially such rest is compelled by pain.

Concussion of the brain, whether accompanied by fracture of the skull or not, usually results in a period of unconsciousness lasting from a minute or so to many weeks. Recovery of consciousness is usually attended by headache and this leads naturally to complete rest in dark and quiet conditions. Too early mobilization, too much noise or use of the eyes may lead to very prolonged disability associated with headaches and giddiness.

Laryngitis often leads to hoarseness due to involvement of the vocal cords, and attempts to speak cause severe pain in the throat. Rest is essential, otherwise prolonged or even permanent damage may occur; once again rest is enforced by pain.

Peritonitis, perhaps due to an inflamed appendix or a perforated ulcer or a penetrating abdominal wound, was an extremely serious condition before modern surgery; yet people with peritonitis *did* recover without operation, and a number still do, even under primitive conditions. The intense pain compels immobility; movements of the bowel itself cease because it is paralysed and any muscular action that would disturb the stillness within the abdominal cavity is prohibited; breathing becomes entirely thoracic because the diaphragm is completely immobilized. The abdominal muscles go into fixed spasm guarding against the smallest movement. In these circumstances the affected coils of bowel can stick together, walling off the appendix, or sealing a perforation. If the shock and infection are not overwhelming repair will occur, possibly with the formation of a localized abscess that will eventually find its way to the surface or rupture into the bowel, thus leading to spontaneous resolution. When we operate on such patients we anticipate and hasten these very processes; we seal perforations, remove inflamed organs, provide drainage tubes, and disturb the rest of the abdominal cavity as little as possible to avoid spreading the infection still further. Indeed if things have already reached the stage of *walling-off infection* we may find it safer not to operate at once but to allow nature to proceed with the localization; many of these patients recover completely from the attack allowing us to remove an appendix or gallbladder easily and safely later on.

These examples are quoted to show that under natural conditions pain has this very definite function of helping repair by compelling rest, and it would be easy to give many more. You will hear it said that the pain of appendicitis (for instance) can have no purpose because surgeons are an extremely recent addition to our evolutionary progress. This view is naïve. Quite obviously the pain of appendicitis was not given us by God for the purpose of enabling surgeons to diagnose the condition, but we have just seen that cases can recover in the absence of surgeons, aided by pain.

I shall try to show later in this part that man is making very considerable use of characteristic pains in the diagnosis of disease and while this cannot in itself be termed a purpose the fact remains that pain has a still wider function in nature—that of *calling attention to trouble*, both the attention of the individual and that of others. Notice that the reactions to pain often include crying, screaming and struggling—displays that invite attention from others. They begin from birth and initially have intrinsic value for the individual in the form of ventilation of the lungs and exercise of the muscles. In fact, if a new-born baby does not cry it may get a slap on the bottom from the midwife or doctor—a fact that some psychiatrists find a little indigestible. The hungry infant cries, screams and struggles, getting attention from its mother and logically a meal; if hunger is in fact the cause the reactions cease with the feeding. Exactly the same reactions can be caused by a strangulated hernia or an inflamed toe or a stabbing nappy pin (the tiny infant seems unable to localize the cause) and we cannot say with certainty that these conditions are painful while mere hunger is not. Relief of the cause will normally bring cessation of the screaming and struggling.

The Cry for Help

The young hurt animal makes a good deal of noise and this usually results in immediate parental investigation. The situation may be resolvable or it may not, but without the cry there is no chance at all.

Now of course help is not always available, and even if the cry is heard maybe nothing can be done. But this is not the fault of the system, and it is hard to imagine anything that could replace an anguished scream as a method of getting help for distress if such help is possible at all – it is primitive and direct and immediate. Perhaps you think this is a 'Wonders of Nature' kind of explanation and implies the facile teleology I am trying to avoid. Well, nature is certainly wonderful by any definition, but she shows no mercy in adversity and no forgiveness for weakness. Is the wounded animal worth saving, or is it a menace to the community? If the latter, its cries may bring predators that will rapidly destroy it. Animals in the wild cannot afford to be burdened with chronic sick or the elderly in pain. Are we upsetting the so-called balance of nature by extending life beyond its 'useful span'? We are only at the beginning of problems in this field; failing kidneys and hearts, blood vessels, livers and lungs are already being replaced by young healthy organs or by artificial ones, in some cases to support failing brains, which will not be replaceable for many years, if ever. Yet progress in this direction is inevitable and certain, and so is progress towards total nuclear war in which individual pain will be of little account, so perhaps some kind of crude balance will be achieved.

Congenital Indifference to Pain

Individuals with this rare anomaly can survive under modern sheltered conditions; otherwise they are at severe risk and seldom live long. They can adapt only if brought up and surrounded by normal sympathetic people. A similar indifference to pain is observed in a special kind of idiocy; occasionally these people deliberately inflict cuts and burns on themselves, appearing to enjoy the sensation. They can only live, for a short time, under the closest institutional care.

The existence of such cases is occasionally quoted to exemplify the uselessness of pain; the argument is shallow and invalid.

The fact that we can sometimes accept painful therapy indicates the vast complexity of our neural pathways. The painful stimulus is not simply conveyed into consciousness as a pain originating in some particular place, but is automatically related to the entire organism, and its past, present and future environment, as well as to our particular social, religious and emotional make-up. We may therefore arrive at the *conscious* decision 'this pain is something that I must bear' and I think it takes an almost human brain to do this. Perhaps not completely human; those who have handled dogs know that they will patiently bear quite a painful procedure if they trust the operator and realize that he is trying to help them.

It would be easy to give hundreds of examples to show that pair has an essential survival value and that we could not exist without it, but perhaps enough has been said to support the point in a general way. We shall now go a stage further and consider ways in which pain is instinctively and naturally *used* by living creatures, particularly ourselves, for further benefit.

Pain as a Means of Defence

Many animals are equipped with the means of inflicting pain on others – horns, claws, teeth, pincers and stings. Most of these may basically be offensive weapons used to obtain food, but anyone who takes liberties with animals or their young knows he risks a quick bite or scratch or sting that warns him not to do it again. Nearly all higher animals instinctively inflict pain as a means of warning or defence, even if they are vegetarians and never kill for food. Some quite delicate creatures are armed with such defensive weapons; think of hedgehogs and porcupines, and of fish that would be instantly devoured by predators were it not for the violent punishment awarded for touching them. An example of this category is the electric eel (*electrophorus electricus*), a South American fresh water fish which occasionally reaches a length of ten feet. Its electric organ consists of highly modified muscle and nerve tissue, forming a battery of closely packed plates, and is capable of delivering a current of 1,000 watts (500 volts, 2 amps) at will—enough to stun a horse or a man and indeed to kill many creatures. At least three other kinds of electric eels or fish exist in different parts of the world, each apparently quite separately evolved.

A very interesting aspect of this defensive use of pain is its employment by *plants*, which themselves do not feel pain (mandrakes notwithstanding), although a simple withdrawal 'reflex' is sometimes seen, as in the sensitive plant (*mimosa pudica*) which flicks its leaves away if they are touched. Many plants are equipped with spikes, thorns and stings for the specific effect of deterring animals from eating them. Who would want a second mouthful of holly? Of course, other creatures evolve with the means of overcoming the deterrent and relish a diet of thistles, but it is this leapfrog overcoming of difficulties that is the essence of evolutionary advance. (The Algerian peasants' trick of eating live scorpions is in a different category.)

Animals seem to know precisely how far they can go without inflicting actual damage, probably the result of the experience gained in play. Two puppies engaged in mock fighting make all the gestures and noises yet on the whole keep the biting below pain level; exceeding this brings a yelp and probably retribution. It is even more fascinating to see the behaviour of a large pet dog with a small child; it tolerates an extraordinary amount of discomfort and even pain, and gets presented with mouthfuls of arms and legs, hardly leaving a tooth mark on the tender skin.

In the animal world deliberate aggression, except for obtaining food, is rare, though there are notable exceptions. The massacres inflicted by foxes on chickens do seem to us like sheer wanton killing; certain animals (the rhinoceros and the killer whale) and fish (the pike) are naturally aggressive in the sense that they tend to attack *anything* whether they are hungry or not, but even so the tendency is to kill quickly and efficiently – the broken neck or torn throat. The example so frequently quoted of 'animal cruelty' is the cat and mouse, but the suffering involved is trivial compared with man's inhumanity to himself and other animals. Most (not all) animals attempt to defend themselves when attacked and many are content with giving the aggressor a sharp lesson in the form of pain that will discourage further attacks. Of course this applies strongly to attacks on a mother with young, and often very great tenacity and courage is displayed by the weaker animal in these circumstances. It is seen in the human species as well, although social evolution brings much more subtle methods of counter-attack and revenge – the latter sometimes delayed for years.

Primitive Education

The second half of this part deals with the ways in which man has adapted and used the sense of pain for benefit to the community as a whole and to the individual. These uses are mainly medical and disciplinary, but before we leave the subject of the natural functions of pain we might notice that a certain rough discipline forms part of the training of many young animals in the wild state. Physical co-ordination occurs very much earlier than it does in men so that the baby animal is capable of running into danger long before it realizes that danger even exists. Parental restraint is applied frequently and forcefully, often with quite painful cuffs and nips, and the infant's reaction of hurt astonishment can be very amusing to watch.

Rough treatment for quite the opposite purpose is seen when the young animal is being forced to take some essential step in its education, usually the moment when it has to face the big outside world on its own for the first time. We observe this behaviour in birds compelling the reluctant fledgling to leave the nest, and in seals forcing their young into the water. The methods of persuasion required may strike us as cruel, but they are an absolute and necessary part of the animal's life history and therefore of the evolutionary process itself.

THE ACCEPTABLE USES OF PAIN

Here I shall try to present some examples of how man has used pain to his advantage in ways that can hardly be considered as part of its biological significance. The two main categories are Diagnostic and Disciplinary.

The Diagnostic Value of Pain

We have already seen how injury or disease in different parts of the body may give rise to particular kinds of pain; it is a logical step to deduce the cause from the effect, and in fact pain is by far the most common and valuable symptom available to physicians for the diagnosis of disease. The medical text-book known as French's *Index of Differential Diagnosis* lists over four hundred items under 'Pain'.

This use of pain is extremely ancient and is seen in every race, however backward. Primitive communities all have their Medicine Man under various names and this individual often occupies a position of authority and power vastly greater than that of his more civilized colleagues. This is largely due to a higher proportion of fear based on superstition than is customary in orthodox medicine, but the need for those in physical distress to seek expert relief is a basic one, so people in pain fly to the Medicine Man.

It must be admitted that the results of most 'witch doctor' treatment compare very unfavourably with those achieved by sheer blind instinct, which usually dictates non-interference and rest. A certain amount of crude psychology is exhibited, the more effective because of the credulous suggestibility of the patient, but on the whole 'witch doctor' medicine is actively harmful, and many a well-meaning medical missionary has been disheartened and defeated by the faith placed in professional opposition of this kind.[1]

Nevertheless the foundations of scientific medicine are implicit in the procedure followed.

1. The patient complains of certain symptoms (pain in the head, vomiting, giddiness).
2. The condition is investigated (casting of little bones, whirling dances, animal sacrifices, etc. etc.).
3. A diagnosis is made (He has a devil in his head).
4. Suitable treatment is given (The patient must make great efforts to expel the devil, so an emetic mixture of dried blood, ground bones and pounded cactus is administered, potentiated by substantial offerings to the tribal gods *via* the High Priest, i.e. the witch doctor).

That in most cases the diagnosis is completely erroneous and the treatment worse than useless cannot hide the fact that a rough logical sequence has been followed. As in any system depending largely upon powerful psychological stimuli, occasional startling cures occur, and failures can be attributed to the intervention of the forces of evil, or the will of the gods, or to the patient's lack of faith. There is still a little *mystique* attached to the practice of medicine, but on the whole people nowadays regard their doctors as ordinary individuals (quite liable to make mistakes) who have vast resources of scientific research available for the diagnosis and treatment of all complaints, and in particular they expect to be relieved of pain.

It soon becomes apparent that the intensity of pain has little relation to the seriousness of the disease causing it; indeed in the case of stones, whether in the urinary tract or elsewhere, it is said that 'little stones like little dogs make the most noise'. A large stone in the kidney, for instance, gets adapted to the shape of its surroundings and settles down to a comfortable life of slow steady growth until it may ultimately destroy the kidney with hardly a twinge to betray its presence. A tiny stone less than one-eighth of an inch across can escape from the kidney and pass into the long narrow tube leading to the bladder (ureter); its passage down the ureter is

[1] *Doctor Against Witch-Doctor*, E. W. Doell.

marked by a series of muscular spasms causing just about the most intense pain met with in the whole of medical practice. It is important to realize that this pain is absolutely unique and diagnostic, so that without any further investigation a surgeon is able to say with some assurance that:

1. The patient has a small stone in his right ureter.
2. It is approximately at the top, or the middle, or the lower end.
3. From the frequency and change in position, that the stone is travelling down and will accordingly probably get through to the outside.

This last point is of great importance, for if the stone sticks in one place blocking the ureter completely, an operation will be necessary to save the kidney from destruction by back-pressure; and if the stone does impact in this way the pain changes its character and becomes *less* severe.

It is curious that pain of such great intensity is caused when this kind of muscular tube contracts against abnormal resistance. We meet it again in the colic due to gallstones, in the intestinal tract, in the ducts of salivary glands and in arteries suddenly blocked with clots. In each case a diagnosis can usually be made on the history of the pain, and in some cases immediate action has to be taken on this alone.

Examples follow of various diseases producing a typical pain complex by which they can be identified with some certainty in the absence of special investigations.

There are three diagnostic aspects of pain to be considered — history, elicited pain and absence of pain.

In the *history* we get our patient's statement about his pain particularly as regards *site*, *type*, *severity*, *frequency* and *duration*. Quite often a firm diagnosis can be made on the history alone, certainly with sufficient accuracy to start treatment while confirmatory investigations are made.

A man of fifty says that while walking uphill he got a sudden intense stabbing pain down the inner side of his left upper arm; it was very frightening, and he had to sit on a wall, feeling breathless, whereupon it eased somewhat. A passing neighbour gave him a lift home.

This man almost certainly had a small coronary thrombosis; the pain originates in the heart muscle itself but is 'referred' to the skin of the arm which is in the same segmental level (page 28). He will be put on complete rest and the diagnosis confirmed by electrocardiograms and other investigations. Notice that rest will do most of the cure, but it must be prolonged.

A woman of forty complains of quite severe attacks of pain just under the front ribs on the right side; the pain is also felt in the back and the right shoulder, and she says it is worse if she eats oily foods like fried fish.

She is very likely indeed to have gallstones, and the initial investigations with a special kind of X-ray will be so directed. Her pain is mainly caused by muscular spasm of the gallbladder and bile ducts, and is felt immediately over the gallbladder itself besides being 'referred' to the back and shoulder. Pending investigations she can immediately be given drugs for relief of spasm and put on a fat-free diet.

In this case the pain tells her to avoid fats—nothing else.

Notice that we may not detect any abnormality whatever in either of these patients when we examine them; the initial diagnosis is likely to be made on the history of pain alone.

A man of sixty-five tells us that he gets severe cramplike pain in his right calf when he walks, it is getting worse and now he can only walk about a hundred yards before rest is essential.

The muscles of his calf are being starved of blood, probably because the arteries in the leg are narrowed or blocked. We may be able to relieve his pain by certain drugs, or by operations of various kinds.

A boy of twelve has agonizing pain in his groin and on examination we find that he has an exquisitely tender testicle on the same side.

This is very likely to be due to a twist of the testicle, thus cutting off its blood supply, and if so operation within a few hours is the only possible way of saving it—if operation is delayed this vital organ will have to be removed. Notice that pain does *nothing* in this case except call for urgent surgical aid – nothing else can be of the slightest use.

One further point in the history of pain, of importance both in diagnosis and treatment, is its tendency to vary. Increasing pain may make an operation urgent; the success of certain treatments, certainly that of analgesic drugs, is gauged by their alleviation of pain.

Elicited Pain

This means that we actually hurt someone in order to find out what is the matter with them; the procedure is a fundamental and absolutely necessary one in the diagnosis of many diseases, and generally takes the form of discovering *tenderness*.

> *A man of thirty gets a generalized abdominal pain and feels sick. Some hours later it moves vaguely over to the right side. When we see him he is fairly comfortable but when his abdomen is carefully and gently pressed all over we find that he is very tender over a small area a few inches above the right groin, and he flinches when this is touched ('guarding').*

This history makes us strongly suspect appendicitis; it could be several other things but the characteristic tenderness confirms the diagnosis and probably indicates an operation as soon as possible.

> *A man of forty has fallen and injured his hand. There is no deformity, but very careful pressure all round the wrist elicits pain in a small area near the base of the thumb.*

This suggests fracture of a small bone (the scaphoid). To avoid prolonged disability a diagnosis should be made early and appropriate treatment given, with a special plaster cast. Evidently a lot depends on elicited pain; in this case it is initially even more important than the X-ray picture, which may show nothing.

> *A young patient has fever and headache, he lies in bed with his head tilted back, and when we try to flex it severe pain is evident.*

This sign suggests *meningitis* at a time when few other signs are positive, and active treatment with antibiotics may be the only hope of saving life.

One could cite pages of examples (French lists two hundred items under 'Tenderness') many of which are everyday experiences. Pain is by far the most common reason for consulting doctors, and the kind of pain, plus various painful manipulations, are his most powerful sources of diagnosis on first contact. It will be appreciated that both sources can take extremely subtle forms, and the obvious diagnosis is not by any means necessarily the correct one. The matter is greatly complicated by a lack of accurate localization as one recedes from the surface of the body, and by the factor of '*referred pain*' by which injury or disease in some part of the body may be felt in another part. We may thus be presented with a patient complaining of pain in his knee, yet find it to be normal on examination and on X-ray. This will lead a more astute clinician to examine the patient's hip, and he may discover evidence of disease there, including local tenderness or pain on extremes of movement.

Other examples of referred pain are tenderness just under the middle of the collar bone, caused by a ruptured intervertebral disc in the lower neck; shooting pains in the trunk and limbs, due to spinal cord involvement in *tabes dorsalis*; and extreme burning pain with exquisite tenderness of the hand and fingers (causalgia) due to compression of the median nerve at some point much higher in the arm. Local treatment of these pains is ineffective, though occasionally soothing. The only chance of cure lies in correct diagnosis by people aware of the possibilities, followed by treatment of the cause. The ability to do this has only been acquired very recently. Most of the causes, however, are a great deal older than Man, who only began to emerge from his primate background about a million years ago. Examination of dinosaur skeletons some hundred million years old shows that their joints were often remarkably arthritic, which must be very trying when you weigh several tons. Almost every bone disease known today can be seen in Stone Age skeletons.

The venerable Pithecanthropus from 500,000 BC had a growth on his femur (thigh bone), and it undoubtedly caused severe pain. We have seen that such pain has always served some function in the protection and evolution of higher creatures, and the fact that Man has only just discovered how to use it in diagnosis is no argument against its place in nature.

It should be mentioned in passing that modern patients accept the necessity for elicited pain when being examined by a doctor so long as it is not too severe. There is in fact no reason to extend this kind of examination beyond brief tolerable limits, but one does find occasionally that a patient with peritonitis has been examined for abdominal tenderness by several different people before the decision to operate is made – by the general practitioner at home, and then by three or four doctors successively at the hospital. If the diagnosis is still in doubt these examinations may be repeated, perhaps adding one by the consultant. The patient with peritonitis and conditions resembling it is in severe pain, but relief in the form of drugs cannot be given until a definite diagnosis has been established, and this may not be at all easy. So none of the above-mentioned doctors dares give morphine until the final decision has been made – to operate or not to operate. A solution of this problem involves a system of highly trained general practitioners referring such cases directly to the operating surgeon – an ideal occasionally realized even today.

August Bier once said that a doctor must cause no pain. Such idealistic statements tend to lose force by their sheer impossibility, but it is certainly necessary for doctors to examine and treat patients with the utmost gentleness at all times, to be constantly aware of the reality of pain. If we modify Bier's words and say that one should never cause or permit unnecessary pain it seems to me we have a precept that could be followed with advantage by the whole of humanity.

Of course this viewpoint is essentially modern. Before the development of anaesthetics and analgesics pain was regarded as inevitable, indeed in some opinions as part of the Divine Plan. The almost ludicrous opposition to the use of chloroform for childbirth is an example of such thinking. What most people do not realize is how very recent the change of attitude is; nowadays anyone suffering more than slight discomfort is encouraged to seek medical advice – it might be something serious. Moreover, with certain exceptions, treatment is not expected to be painful, though some discomfort is anticipated after most operations. As late as 1840 the treatment of many diseases was known to be so violently painful that they were allowed to reach the stage of agony before medical help was sought, and by then the cause was usually easily diagnosed. I should like to cite the case of a stone in the urinary bladder as an example of this and many other points raised in this book.

The Awful History of Bladder Stones

This condition is probably as old as Man, and no race is exempt. Dietary indiscretions and the prevalence of bladder infection (cystitis) resulted in a greatly increased incidence in the past, particularly in male children, and it is still common in backward communities. Without going deeply into causative theories, what happens is this: a deposit of crystals occurs around a tiny abnormality in the bladder wall, and this grows by the deposit of successive layers until it reaches a size too large for passage through the narrow urethra to the outside. Later it becomes detached and lies loose in the bladder. During this process various small pieces known as 'gravel' may be passed, but the stone itself may grow to a diameter of several centimetres. So long as the bladder contains urine and is filling slowly nothing is felt, but a point is reached when the desire to pass water is experienced and later becomes urgent.

The act of micturition is complex. Normally it is initiated voluntarily, then it becomes automatic with relaxation of the sphincter muscle guarding the outlet and powerful contraction of the muscular wall of the bladder itself until it is completely emptied. Now the lining membrane of the bladder is normally quite insensitive except in a small area near the exit (the *trigone*) which is exquisitely sensitive. Also, contractions of the muscular wall are not felt unless they are against abnormal resistance, as in obstruction to the outflow, when great pain is experienced. If the bladder contains a stone micturition proceeds normally until nearly the end, then the stone drops into the *trigone* area and blocks the outlet. Excruciating sudden pain occurs from contact of the rough surface with the *trigone*, and very intense contraction of the muscles endeavouring ineffectually to expel the stone – a process often leading to bleeding in the water. The pain is felt centrally just above the pubic bone, and in the male is referred down to the end of the penis. (Most cases are males because the urethra is much narrower.) At a later stage infection

occurs and then the whole of the inside of the bladder is also
sensitive to pain.

The adult with this condition may learn a certain amount of
control so that his bladder is only partially emptied, but the child
finds it very difficult to stop once he has started. The plight of the
small boy with a bladder stone was pitiful in the extreme. Terrified
of the consequences, he held his water until the sheer bursting pain
forced him to let go, and then he got the full agonizing pain at the
end. Some of these boys used to clutch and pull at their penis in a
frantic attempt to ease it, bringing accusations of masturbation; the
'treatment' for this included beating, and blistering or cauterizing
the thighs or even the penis itself.[1] It is difficult to see any biological significance in such events, and I think the only possible
answer is that in the human species there are none. Under extremely
primitive conditions it might result in the elimination of a weak
member of the community, but once the stone has reached a certain
size it cannot be passed or removed without surgical intervention
and all the suffering is useless.

The diagnosis *was* sometimes made, in primitive societies, on
grounds of the typical pain, bleeding, the passage of gravel and the
swollen bladder above the pubic bone. Occasional efforts were made
to get at the stone by plunging a knife into the bladder and no doubt
some of these were successful. The patient's condition afterwards
was however even worse than before; he either got peritonitis and
died, or he acquired a permanent painful ulcerating urinary leak
with eventual death from infection. Operations to remove these
stones were done long before anaesthesia was invented; some are
recorded by the Greek surgeon Celsus in AD 50, and successful
operations were undoubtedly performed by the Indian surgeon
Susutra, in the fifth century AD. Once the anatomy was better
understood an approach was planned that avoided peritonitis and
carried much less risk of subsequent leaking. This required the
patient lying on his back with his legs flexed, and the insertion of a
knife between the anus and the genitalia just to one side (this position

---

[1] Perhaps you think that this was only done by ignorant or sadistic people. Not so.
One of the greatest surgeons of the last century was John Hilton, to whom I have
already referred in connection with his lectures on 'Rest and Pain'. Hilton recommended blistering the penis with iodine for 'onanism', and treated both adults and
children in this way for at least twenty years of his active life.

is still known as the *lithotomy* or 'cutting for stone' position); the object was to feel the stone with the point of the knife at a depth of about three to four inches, then to seize it with a long forceps and drag it out, preferably intact.

It is hardly necessary to point out that this process was extremely painful, and put a premium on sheer speed. It was essential to strap the patient very tightly in position to avoid movement, and it took a great deal of practice and skill to hit the stone quickly. Lithotomists who could do the whole job in a few minutes were in great demand. The St Thomas's Hospital surgeon William Cheselden often did it in one minute (his record was fifty-four seconds), in the eighteenth century, and in the end he contented himself with four or five operations a year at £500 a time – roughly equivalent to £5,000 today. Even at this speed the time of suffering must have seemed an eternity, and people put up with years of violent pain before finally nerving themselves to face the ordeal of surgery. (One sufferer from bladder stone was Samuel Pepys, and another was the notorious Judge Jefferies, who conducted the Bloody Assizes in 1685.)

The average maximum operating time for bladder stone by competent surgeons in the early nineteenth century was six minutes. There was a very unfortunate case at Guy's Hospital in 1828. Bransby Cooper, nephew of the great Sir Astley Cooper, ran into difficulties, and after twenty minutes of unsuccessful cutting and probing cried 'Give me my uncle's knife!' Regrettably this notable instrument failed to improve matters, and it took Bransby another thirty-five minutes to produce the stone. The exhausted patient died the next day. Following this episode a lengthy and vituperative article appeared in the *Lancet* (now perhaps the most ethical of all medical journals) in which it was suggested that Bransby Cooper was an 'incompetent bungler' against whom the public should be protected, and further that he had been appointed Surgeon to Guy's by a 'gang' simply because he was Sir Astley's nephew. A tremendous libel action resulted, heard in a crowded court. Among the witnesses were the young John Hilton and Dr Roget of subsequent Thesaurus fame. Bransby Cooper got the verdict and was awarded £100 damages. The case caused enormous public interest, and numerous newspapers published witty articles and cartoons.

It was during this period that clinical diagnostic skill reached its highest peak, lacking X-rays and other scientific aids, and carrying the absolute necessity to avoid surgery if possible. Very great reliance was placed upon precise observations of the type, duration, severity and location of pain, and this pioneer work remains the basis of present-day medicine.

Absence of Pain

There is a tendency for people to disregard personal abnormalities if they do not hurt; we may thus be presented with an inoperable cancer of the breast which has been allowed to develop over a period of two years or more because there was no pain. This painlessness has diagnostic significance in many cases and therefore may influence the whole course of treatment. Examples are the deepening painless jaundice from growths in the bile ducts (stones are usually painful); the painless destruction of joints in certain kinds of syphilitic disease; and the 'glove and stocking' distribution of anaesthesia characteristic of hysteria. The exact shape of an area of skin numbness can be mapped out by the simple use of a pin, and this will enable a neurologist to state the nerves affected, the precise level of their involvement, and often the kind of disease to be expected. In fact, the complete absence of pain automatically eliminates a number of causes, and suggests others, for any particular disability.

Further Medical Uses of Pain

Occasionally a deep dull distressing pain can be alleviated by substituting a sharper but more tolerable superficial one (see Counter-irritation, page 124). In less enlightened days red-hot irons were used with horrifying frequency and doubtless served the purpose of diverting attention from the patient's original complaint.

A more recent example is the employment of painful stimuli in *aversion therapy*; the unfortunate patient is shown photographs and films of his favourite obsession (homosexuality, gambling) but the

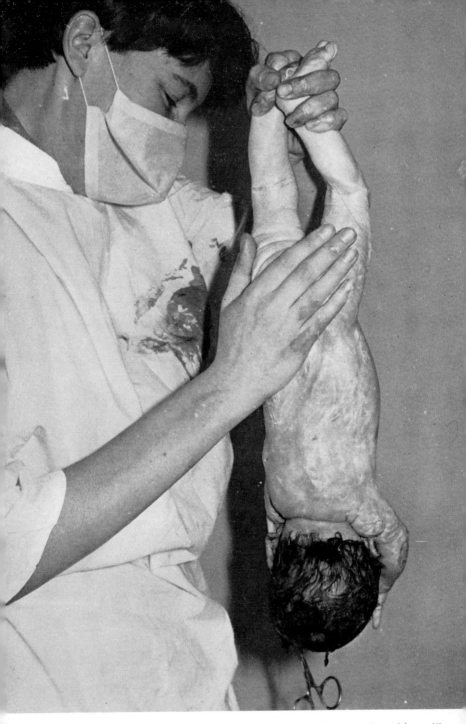

Introduction to pain. Slapping a new-born baby to make it start breathing. (See
49) *Photo: Richard Serjeant*

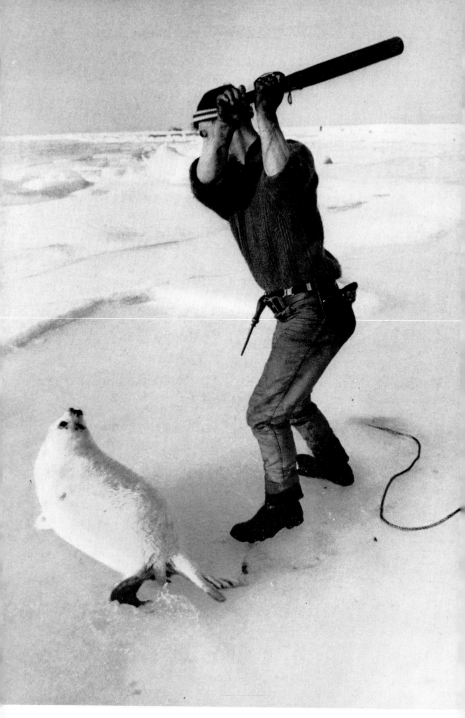

2 Sealskin coat at an early stage of production. The man's licence costs one do
(See p. 89) *Photo: Syndication International*

show is spoiled by giving him painful electric shocks, or making him violently sick with a drug called apomorphine, at the most interesting moments. The method has not received unanimous approval from the psychiatric fraternity, mainly because it appears to lack the finer theoretical *nuances*, but some spectacular successes are claimed.

Discipline

The principle of 'punishment for wrong' must be at least as old as Man, probably far older: 'reward for right' as an addition certainly came much later, and as an alternative is still struggling.

In the grim hostile world of primitive society Man can have had no time for kindness; cuffs, blows and severe punishments were the only means of dissuading dependants from foolhardy actions and enforcing essential learning. Survival proves their efficacy. It is hardly surprising that the impulse to hurt the child who makes dangerous experiments is instinctive, particularly if they are anti-social, and within certain limits such action is accepted by the child as being just. In the fullness of time we shall doubtless reach a stage where any kind of corporal punishment is unthinkable, but there will have to be a very satisfactory alternative to the quick slap for some kinds of misbehaviour. Enlightened intelligent parents in comfortable circumstances can often bring up a small family without 'raising a hand against them in anger', but the vast majority of people do not belong to this group. Many are ignorant and stupid and try to bring up large families in a squalid sordid environment. If their children are to cope with this kind of life, or even escape from it, they may have to learn the hard way, and this involves pain.

There can be few parents who have not encountered deliberately challenging defiance on the part of a child, usually on some fairly trivial matter like putting on a macintosh before going out in the rain. After due warnings instructions are ignored and in comes Percy soaked to the skin. Stripping, drying and reclothing are accompanied by expressions of displeasure and the warning: 'If you do that again you will get a hard slap.' Half an hour later Percy is found outside with another set of soaked garments.

3

Now this is a situation calling for action, an action the parent must win, or lose face. If the slap has been threatened and defiance exhibited, the slap must be given. Most parents would know precisely how hard, too; hard enough to hurt, but not to damage; to deter, but not to humiliate.

It is probably true to say that a quick hard slap on the backside, given immediately after due warning, and merited by some obvious default, is recognized by children as being just and accordingly *not* resented and *not* used as a basis for some later complex. It will most certainly do less harm than prolonged curtailment of liberty, or expressions like 'Mummy won't love you if you do that'. Part of nature's programme is to fit the young animal for the environment he will later have to cope with alone, and her methods of doing so do not include psychotherapy or the Welfare State. 'Rough justice' implies pain, but it also specifies justice: young children seem to have an acute sense of what is just and fair, and if cuffs and slaps or even thrashings are a common part of the environment they will be accepted by the child as part of life. In fact, parents lacking the benefits of modern sociological and psychiatric guidance (99.999 per cent of parents) will use instinctive methods, and these certainly include the quick slap.

The big trouble with this system is that it leads imperceptibly into viciousness and cruelty. However well-merited the blow, the discerning and self-critical donor will usually regret it and wish some other way had been possible.

Training Animals

All animal training, whether for work or for public exhibition, is conducted on the basic principle of punishment and reward. Sometimes there is more of one than the other and one could quote a great many examples of the utmost cruelty used for both these purposes. There is, however, a basic difference between flogging a wild horse to break it in and the pain inflicted on a tiger for public exhibition in a circus. Training animals for work may well be essential to the life of a community; although complete callousness is often evident, much of it is due to sheer ignorance, and in most cases the animal is too valuable to be killed or incapacitated in the process.

Perhaps in the ideal world there would be no disease, no necessity for punishment; all training would be done by kindness, and all misfits rehabilitated. We are very far from realizing such conditions, and until we do pain will continue to play an essential part in our lives. At present its place in Medicine is integral and necessary; with discipline of children we are on less certain grounds, especially in highly civilized societies, but it is widely used and in minor degrees probably does less harm than most alternatives. A few countries do however seem to have arrived at a stage of civilization when all other forms of deliberately inflicted pain are unjustifiable on any grounds.

PART THREE

PROBLEMS AND PENALTIES

PROBLEMS

THERE IS NO real difficulty in accounting for moderate degrees of pain, or even in justifying its use for a number of purposes not directly connected with its biological significance. It is when pain becomes agony that problems arise – not only about its very existence but also about Man's readiness to inflict it, and on occasion his capacity to endure it.

Any attempt to consider these problems objectively must begin with the fundamental question – why does extreme pain exist at all?

It must be admitted that a purely scientific approach to this question is not very rewarding, and apart from the function of agony in nature in calling attention to the hopelessly injured and their subsequent destruction, explanation is lacking. Philosophical approaches with a powerful religious bias carry even less weight, mainly because the biological aspects are ignored and the entire phenomenon is regarded as a kind of heavenly immigration clearance, under which one must be forgiven for visualizing a Pain Officer whose task would be to assess the precise degree of individual suffering.

There seems no purpose or use for the intense sensitivity of the nail beds, or the torments that result from an impacted ureteric stone; moderately severe pain should be enough. In fact people without a sense of pain at all (those with the very rare condition known as 'congenital indifference to pain') are sometimes able to adapt to a fairly normal existence provided that they are reasonably intelligent and are looked after by people with normal senses.

Practically any part of the body can be stimulated to the point of intolerable pain, indeed to the point of loss of all control and at least temporary insanity. On general grounds it seems unlikely that sensations of such enormous power should be mere by-products of complex nervous systems, without intrinsic biological significance; one feels certain that the ruthless selection of the evolutionary process must have used agony as one of the prices of survival — violent sensation calling for violent action — and presumably the less punishing devices had been tried and found wanting. Of course the whole of nature is a fantastic compromise, nothing in itself being perfect; but sometimes the price does seems very high.

Abnormally low reactions to pain may characterize certain individuals through the whole range of possible stimuli, and a few of these may be among the rare people who succeed in enduring torture over long periods without giving way.

Cruelty may be defined as the infliction or permission of unnecessary pain, in the knowledge that suffering is thereby caused. *Sadism* is a special form of cruelty in which a sexual element predominates. *Masochism* is a sexual form of enjoyment of pain, but there is no specific term for the much more common enjoyment of minor degrees of pain with a non-sexual basis.

A good deal of what follows refers to pain in animals, so perhaps we had better clarify a point or two about this first.

Every particle of factual evidence supports the contention that the higher mammalian vertebrates experience pain sensations at least as acute as our own. To say that they feel less because they are lower animals is an absurdity; it can easily be shown that many of their senses are far more acute than ours — visual acuity in certain birds, hearing in most wild animals, and touch in others; these animals depend more than we do today on the sharpest possible awareness of a hostile environment. Apart from the complexity of the cerebral cortex (which does not directly perceive pain) their nervous systems are almost identical to ours and their reactions to pain remarkably similar, though lacking (so far as we know) the philosophical and moral overtones. The emotional element is all too evident, mainly in the form of fear and anger. In countries where ill-treatment of animals is commonplace (most countries) the argument is often advanced that it doesn't matter, because they have no souls. Ignoring the arrogant stupidity of this we shall assume that such animals feel pain much as we do, and that it does matter.

THE INGREDIENTS OF CRUELTY

The search for reasons behind ultimates in human behaviour is rather like the pursuit of fundamental particles in atomic physics. The first step beyond Dalton seemed final – matter consisted of protons and electrons. Inconsistencies crept in, and neutrons were added. Later it became necessary to postulate mesons and neutrinos; all these particles are found to have corresponding anti-particles, doubling their number. At the time of writing there are over a hundred 'fundamental' particles, some with curious properties such as absence of mass. We now have the half-jocular hypothesis of 'Quarks' (and even anti-Quark) whose main feature appears to be the impossibility that they can ever be observed.

Thus in human behaviour the ultimate breakdown has been said in the past to be pleasure and pain: but there are so many aspects of this – sex, hate, love, vengeance, faith and so on, which seem to resist breakdown – and why not? Surely an animal is more complex than its component atoms. Let us look at some of the 'fundamental particles' leading to cruelty and violence, bearing in mind that they overlap to a very large extent and are rarely alone as motives.

The main ingredients of cruelty are callousness, ignorance, power in the hands of psychopaths, fear, intolerance, hate, vengeance, avarice, superstition, and perversions of sex. Almost every act of cruelty contains elements of these, alone or in various combinations. These are fairly obvious ones, but there are cases almost beyond reasonable analysis, with motives too deep for conscious realization.

Probably at normal times the majority of people in any community dislike giving or receiving pain, and are on the whole only too happy if they can be left in peace to work and play in harmony with their neighbours. Unfortunately Man has seldom been allowed to do these things by his rulers and those who make themselves responsible for enforcing his spiritual views, and it was easier in the past for nuclei of tyranny and intolerance to thrive, with consequent inevitable cruelty. Once such a system becomes established and backed by power there is very little the average inoffensive citizen can do about it – he has to accept it as part of the only life he knows, and try to keep out of trouble; and in these circumstances trouble means pain.

Surrounded with constant pain associated with disease and with punishment the development of individual callousness follows, mainly because any non-conformity marks the man as being either soft or dangerous. This armour of callousness influences the man's total attitude, particularly towards those weaker than himself – his servants, his animals, even his own children, and particularly towards those he has been taught to regard as criminals, enemies, or inferior beings.

Ignorance and *Curiosity* sometimes go together, as when a young child torments some animal without any conscious desire to cause pain – he is trying to find out what happens. A good deal of pain is caused because people simply do not realize how painful some procedures are; perhaps they themselves have a high tolerance or have no personal experience of bad pain. Doctors, dentists and nurses need to be very careful in this respect, because of the things they have to do, and unfortunately one occasionally sees quite unnecessary suffering caused by thoughtless behaviour.

Power in the hands of psychopaths is one of the most dangerous influences in the world. It leads in minor degrees to tyrannies and bullying in homes, schools, factories, the armed forces, and many other places. At extremes it places bodies and lives in the hands of madmen, to do with as they will, and we shall see examples of what can happen.

Vengeance is an almost instinctive emotion and one encouraged by the Old Testament – Jehovah was a great one for revenge. One of the difficulties of judicial systems is to make them rational and not based on the desire of the wronged party for vengeance. Vicious systems have always been supported by the masses, exemplified by the popularity of public executions and punishments. Vengeance is expressed through pain in so many ways that it would take volumes to name them. They range from whipping a troublesome dog to the massacre of whole populations with every possible variety and refinement of cruelty.

Superstition

> *Never tilt against the ruling superstition,*
> *unless you be powerful enough to withstand*
> *it, or clever enough to escape its pursuit.*
>
> VOLTAIRE

Superstition is a religion or belief based on credulity and fear, and sometimes there is great difficulty in distinguishing between this and other kinds of religion. It leads to excesses like those of the Inquisition, ritual torture for the purpose of obtaining rain during dry periods in almost all primitive societies, and persecution on a wholesale scale as seen very recently.

The Massacre of the Innocents by Herod was motivated by superstition and fear; perhaps less well-known (but better authenticated) is that European parents used to flog their children in bed on Innocents' Day — a practice that persisted until the seventeenth century. In England children were also regularly beaten by their parents on the occasion of public hangings.

Infanticide was quite common in primitive societies, especially for abnormalities such as accessory fingers or even for breech presentations at birth. In Hawaii it was usual to kill all children after the fourth by burying them alive in cow-dung.

Belief in *Sorcery and Witchcraft* is as old as the power to believe, and all these activities were severely dealt with in the ancient world. The subject is dealt with further on page 109.

Initiation Ceremonies have always been the excuse for a great deal of sadistic behaviour, with sexual instruction of the utmost crudity and barbarities such as female circumcision and infibulation; these were certainly practised in Egypt, Arabia, Ethiopia, Persia, Australia and Africa. Even so, the initiation rites have two basic purposes — sexual instruction for the young and the lesson that pain must be endured. We appear to be still struggling in both of these fields.

There exists quite widely a view that pain's purpose is that of a test of character, a kind of portal to various rewards. Probably nobody's view of life is complete without experiencing pain in some form; otherwise such a view is incomplete and likely to be unsympathetic. Nevertheless one makes mental reservations about this, particularly regarding the amount of pain necessary to induce such understanding, and it may be felt that comprehension of the various problems can be reached without being blinded with red-hot irons or having one's testicles crushed between stones.

Is it necessary to suffer in order to obtain salvation? If so, how much? For every martyr, thousands of innocent people renounced their faith, confessed to ludicrous things and were reduced to gibbering lunatics. Does this justify pain?

In the lay hierarchy of the Christian heaven the 'noble army of martyrs' stands third in order of precedence—after the Apostles and the Prophets. Martyrdom is therefore the ordinary man's only means of entry, and a very hard way indeed, as reference to Fox or Galloni[1] will show. If the divine purpose of agony is to provide martyrs it seems remarkably wasteful, not only in human beings but in the whole of evolution leading to them, and also a little rough on those whose views, tenacity and opportunities do not fit for such office. It must however be remembered that economy is not characteristic of natural processes, rather extreme prodigality; if the system is compared with the wastage of human spermatozoa (approximately 500,000 million to a single live birth), or with the immense mortality of elvers in the life history of eels, it is not completely out of proportion.

All religions (unless atheism is included) postulate superior beings who are interested in human activities and can be persuaded by suitable approaches to alter the arrangements that they have made.

It is sometimes said that in view of the ultra-microscopic size of the earth in relation to the universe (or even to our own galaxy, which contains 100,000 million stars) any gods whose main interest is in the human race must be very little gods. This argument is not very impressive. Assuming we do not terminate the whole process with some senseless atom war, the technical advances in the next five million years or so, together with an increase of population at

---

[1] *The Acts and Monuments of Martyrs*, Fox; *Tortures and Torments of the Christian Martyrs*, Galloni; Joseph McCabe, in his book, *The Popes and Their Church*, refers to these works as 'impudent forgeries', and of course they contain much highly biased fiction. They nevertheless reflect the customs and tendencies of their period.

roughly the present rate, should enable us to colonize a fair proportion of the planets in the galaxy. It seems more than likely that there are also other contenders in such a field, and perhaps all the pitiful wrigglings we exhibit at the present time are under observation in a manner rather similar to our own technique with experimental animals.

So far as sin is concerned, the great religions of the East incorporate the more logical doctrine of Karma, a man's future being determined by his behaviour and not by cajolery. All religions promise some future life, and all assume that certain men are able by various disciplines to gain direct knowledge of higher states of existence – these men are the priests, adepts, saints and so on. Such beliefs are characteristic of primitive superstitions, Greek mythology, Buddhism, Roman Catholicism and most other faiths.

The people who cross their fingers on seeing a black cat exemplify one basic menace to the survival of Man – a belief in magic. Consciously or unconsciously they are trying to protect themselves against the forces of evil by means of a magic sign. The cat represents the devil, the cross represents crucifixion. Our ancestors in fact used to crucify cats or burn them to death for this very purpose.

Anyone who thinks this is far-fetched should devote a little time to study of *The Golden Bough*.[1] It contains endless examples of insensate cruelty to animals and humans – men, women and children – for the express purpose of placating, propitiating and cajoling gods and spirits. After a lifetime of deep study Frazer concludes that the most powerful forces in the making of religions are *fear of the dead* and *belief in the efficacy of magic*. He further states that such beliefs are invariably held by the dull, the weak, the ignorant and the superstitious – by far the greatest number of people in the world. He refers to 'the solid layer of savagery beneath the surface, unaffected by superficial changes in religion or culture'.

Factors of this kind resulted in the sacrifice of children to Moloch, in roasting people alive in the brazen bull of Minos, in burning animals and people to death in huge wicker baskets by the Druids, in the use of 'scapegoats' throughout history to die painfully as offerings to gods or spirits, and in thousands of other atrocities. The

[1] *The Golden Bough*, Sir James George Frazer, F.R.S.

one common factor in all religions seems to be the persistence of this inner craving for (or fear of) magic. The young child grows up to a world of wonder, and his credulity is fostered with fascinating stories of gnomes, pixies, fairies, talking animals, trolls, giants, wizards and all the rest. It is sometimes very obviously a bitter disappointment to a child to discover that these things are not actually true—a discovery occasionally resulting in scornful scepticism; usually there is insidious substitution by the more subtle magic of superstition or religion, and the intensity with which a man adopts his particular faith depends among many factors on early environmental enthusiasm. The doctrine of sin in some form is invariable, and the hold of religion is tightened by ritual.

At a certain level men may be guided into admirable codes of conduct, and if enlightened recognize the essential similarity of all religions. Unfortunately there is a tendency towards credulity, intellectual enslavement, gross narrowness of outlook, and an awful growth of intolerance—which probably implies the fear that one's faith may be false. Frazer refers to 'the disintegrating forces of religious dissension'. We have already seen examples of the enormities committed in the name of gods; they could be multiplied indefinitely, but the point here is to try and understand the immense hold that a particular set of beliefs can have on a man, a hold far beyond anything the average modern English churchgoer can imagine. And this same burning zeal is capable of carrying people through the barbarities committed by their brethren.

As soon as a religion tries to become rational and 'down to earth' it tends to lose its hold. People drifting away from a boring or routine religion sometimes show their craving for magic by adopting other beliefs with magic attributes—it does not matter how irrational they are so long as they cannot actually be disproved. Most superstitions probably arise in this way and they are by no means confined to the times when priests had a monopoly of education.

One of the most remarkable examples of superstition and magic was the craze for *Spiritualism*, which began in 1847 when two little American sisters named Fox played tricks on their parents and others by producing raps and bangs around the house, promptly interpreted by the grown-ups as being supernatural. The sisters went on doing this for the next forty years, and the cult spread all over Europe. The most elementary conjuring was used by 'mediums' to produce abjectly trivial manifestations and 'voices from the spirit world', mostly in total darkness. One might imagine that this kind of thing would only appeal to credulous, simple and ignorant people. Credulous, yes; simple and ignorant – hardly. Among the ardent supporters and believers in spiritualism were Sir William Crooks (chemist), William McDougall (Harvard psychologist), Sir William Barrett (physicist), Sir Oliver Lodge (physicist), Augustus De Morgan (mathematician), Alfred Russell Wallace (biologist) and Henry Sidgwick (Professor of Moral Philosophy at Cambridge). The last-named founded the Society for Psychical Research.

In America J. F. Rinn and Harry Houdini[1] spent years investigating, exposing, imitating and outclassing mediums. All the famous mediums were eventually exposed in trickery; but the performances continued until the revelations of infra-red photography finally ended any 'physical manifestations',[2] and the less colourful simple messages from the other side are all that remain of a comparatively forgotten cult.

It is very evident from any study of spiritualism that what counted was not the messages but the medium, who made magic of a kind that could be shared by sitting in a circle in the dark and conjuring up strange powers, like the half-forgotten wizards and fairies from childhood. The modern counterpart is the pseudoscience of parapsychology – now I think on the wane. An enormous amount of money and time has been wasted in conducting childish guessing games to try and prove the existence of telepathy and clairvoyance (and even telekinesis) with a complete absence of elementary method that appals the ordinary scientist. It would be a very bold man who denied the existence of telepathy, but on general scientific grounds it is an extremely improbable phenomenon, and proof cannot be obtained by procedures like this. Why has the matter then received so much attention resulting in the establishment of university chairs, the publication of dozens of books and articles and fomented the hottest controversy? Because most people *want* to believe in

---

[1] *Searchlight on Psychical Research*, J. F. Rinn and Harry Houdini.
[2] *The Hand of Mary Constable*, Paul Gallico. This book discloses one method of producing the famous 'wax glove'.

magic, or are afraid of it. The success of Freemasonry depends less on the admirable precepts of brotherhood and fidelity, and the alleged social and business advantages, than on secret signs, obscure ritual, and initiation ceremonies – magic.

Consider also the world-wide interest in Christian Science, and its pitifully inadequate foundations; the fantastic structure of Theosophy and the character of its originators; the vast support for evangelists and revivalists, even in this comparatively sceptical country – people whose message, when analysed in cold print, is often meaningless or puerile. All illustrate the hunger for magic that will lighten dull lives, bolster personal inadequacies, provide apparent meaning where this is lacking, and make some people feel just a little superior to some others.

These are not arguments for atheism, which can be as bigoted as any religion; there is no attempt to deny that higher powers exist, or that for vast numbers of people the belief in them results in widespread charity and self-sacrifice, as well as in personal solace and comfort. Man's difficulty is to find or even imagine a religion worth the name that combines these features with the preservation of an open mind and tolerance for other people's views. The opposites – the closed mind, credulity and intolerance, are without doubt the cause of a vast amount of suffering. The kind of religion based on deception does much more harm than good. It offers escape from responsibilities, entertainment, and social intercourse; it often provides a sublimation for sexuality; it promises marvels to come for the faithful, and dire punishments for backsliders; it usually has facile explanations for pain, totally inadequate when pain comes.

It is certain that in a multitude of cases faith has suffered shipwreck on the rock of meaningless pain.[1]

The amount of pain deliberately inflicted as a direct result of superstition is beyond all calculation; clearly this is one of our fundamental particles.

Many attempts have of course been made by the major religions and philosophers to explain the metaphysics of pain. The Buddhists

[1] *Encyclopaedia of Religion and Ethics*, T. and T. Clarke.

and Schopenhauer seem to adopt the view that life is not important and escape is essential – the pessimistic attitude. The Stoics felt that pain was there to be fought. (Flaubert called Stoicism 'the sublimest kind of stupidity'.) Christian Science implies that pain only exists in the imagination of non-believers, although Mrs Mary Baker Eddy, who founded the cult, flew to her dentist at the slightest touch of toothache. It is hard to imagine a more flagrant misuse of the word 'science'.

The Christian religion puts a premium on the virtue of endurance. The philosophy is approximately that in a sinful world the perfection of souls can be attained by suffering, which is therefore a virtue, but the relief offered by modern drugs and other methods is fully accepted, which leads to some rather muddled thinking.

Mob Violence

Rule based on superstition and bigotry and enforced by any form of dictatorship inevitably leads to persecution and cruelty, often eventually to revolt and wholesale bloodshed.

It would be only too easy to multiply authentic incidents of awful cruelty – indeed many books have been filled with these. Enough has been said to exemplify Man's ingenuity in this respect but perhaps not enough to prove beyond doubt that given the excuse and the opportunity he will revert to such behaviour with enthusiasm. A few examples based on the recorded actions of mobs or systems may lend weight to the point. There is no indication whatever of any lessening of this tendency, though it is kept underground by the more enlightened systems of government.

Genghis Khan is said to have been responsible for the slaughter of at least 1,700,000 people at Mishapur in 1269; the Poles massacred over a hundred thousand Muscovites in 1611, and so forth.

It may be objected that these are things of the past, and anyway exaggerated, so consider some more recent events in which details are available in the form of eye-witness accounts and photographs.

The Austro-Hungarian invasion of Serbia in 1916 was marked

by cruelty equalling anything in history. At least 3,500 civilians were tortured and killed in the parish of Prnjavor alone, 122 being burned alive.[1]

The events in the Red revolution in Russia between 1918 and 1922 show that the Cheka practised flayings and burnings and numerous other primitive tortures on a vast scale, using dungeons reminiscent of the Middle Ages.[2]

In the U.S.A. between 1889 and 1930 official records show that 3,724 persons were lynched, four-fifths of them Negroes, by methods that included man-hunting, mutilations and burning alive. The lynch-mobs had at least 75,000 members, including children. I feel sure most people would say that all the Negroes had raped white women, but in sober statistical fact rape was a factor in only four per cent of cases. For all these killings forty-nine people were indicted, and four sentenced.[3]

The treatment of completely innocent citizens in China by the Japanese in 1937 is hard to believe until one sees, as I have, hundreds of photographs taken at great personal risk with a concealed Leica during the invasion of Nanking. A few such pictures have appeared in books and journals, but no editor would dare to publish most of the obscene atrocities; the people who escaped with a simple beheading were very fortunate indeed.[4]

The Nazi régime was responsible for the death of at least six million Jews, mostly in degrading circumstances, and the amount of pain deliberately inflicted is beyond estimate. The fact that a great deal of this maltreatment was carried out in public, if not with approval certainly without protest from the onlookers, is a grim reminder of how masses can be swayed by certain ideas, no matter how fatuous, to the point of sheer hysteria. Since then we have seen many examples of slaughter, torture and rape in the Congo and other emergent countries, and many seem to be on the brink of such events.

---

[1] *The First Hungarian Invasion of Serbia*, R. A. Reiss, D.Sc.
[2] *The Red Terror in Russia*, S. P. Melgounov.
[3] *The Tragedy of Lynching*, A. F. Raper.
[4] *What War Means*, H. J. Timperley.

Sadism

Some authorities, following Freud, would say that all cruelty has a sexual basis, but since they postulate the same basis for every aspect of human activity their case is not very convincing. At the same time a little analysis does disclose a sexual component in a good deal of cruelty, sometimes not immediately obvious. The term itself is derived from the Marquis de Sade[1] (1740–1814) who was condemned to death at Aix for unnatural offences at the age of thirty-two. He escaped from prison, but was eventually re-tried and confined in the Bastille, where he wrote a large number of plays and obscene novels. He was finally transferred to the Charenton Lunatic Asylum as being incurable, and died there after eleven years in 1814. De Sade was in fact rather a pitiful figure. His actual performances included a few wild parties and a single episode (for which he was convicted) in which he whipped a prostitute, who eventually did very well out of it financially. His books *Justine* and *Juliette* are sheer imaginative pornography without any literary merit, and hence still command excellent sales in Soho. Books of this kind were extremely common at the time, but de Sade's efforts (nearly all written in prison) were exceptional both in volume and content. He wrote at least twenty-two books and fifteen plays, all on roughly the same lines, and the one that got him into real trouble was a scurrilous attack on Napoleon. During the French Revolution he was an advocate of moderation, and denounced capital punishment.

The pure sadist is rare, as one who can only reach sexual satisfaction by the exhibition of cruelty. There are in fact a number of records of men (and women) having orgasms while torturing another person or an animal. In ancient Rome sexual orgies were often accompanied by spectacles of torturing prisoners or slaves. A certain amount of violence is quite common during mating in animals, especially in the cat tribe, and it also occurs during normal human intercourse at times. The tendency towards sadism is exemplified by the invariable acts of rape that accompany mass violence all over the world and by prevalence of sexual assaults on children, sometimes ending in murder.

A great deal of sensational pornographic literature is based on

[1] *The Marquis de Sade, his Life and Works*, G. R. Dawes.

sexual aspects of cruelty; whether these works encourage and inflame such tendencies in their readers is a matter debated with significant heat in relation to censorship, a number of books thus getting read that would otherwise sink into obscurity from sheer triviality or monumental dullness. Every so often action certainly has to be taken, as in the case of the 'horror comics' that sold in millions a few years ago, mainly to the sexually underprivileged. Quite apart from their sadistic subject-matter these publications reached the absolute nadir of literary rubbish, and not even the well-known champions of printed freedom raised a voice in their defence.

De Sade's activities were trivial compared with a number of other characters throughout history. Notorious in the ancient world were the Roman Emperors Caligula, Tiberius and Nero. Since then two men are perhaps worthy of special mention; Gilles de Rais in the Middle Ages, and Peter Kurten in the present century.

Gilles de Rais (1404–1440) was rich, aristocratic and cultured; he was made a Maréchal of France at the age of twenty-five. Disliking women intensely after a disastrous marriage at sixteen, he developed a passion for alchemy and a sadistic obsession for young boys. He and his minions lured the children into the Château de Tiffauges on various pretexts, then assaulted them and tortured them to death in complex and prolonged sessions. These activities went on for nearly eight years, and there is no doubt that the total number of his victims greatly exceeded the one-hundred-and-forty to which he confessed at his trial, each carefully recorded in detail. It seems almost incredible that after sentence he pleaded for absolution and that this was granted.

He was hanged and burned (in that order) on the 26th October 1440, after a fantastic procession which included the Bishop who had tried him; indeed, 'the morning of his execution saw the extraordinary spectacle of the clergy, followed by the entire population of Nantes, who had been clamouring for his death, marching through the streets singing and praying for his salvation'.[1]

Gilles de Rais is perhaps unique, but this is because he had unrivalled opportunities and not because such tendencies are themselves rare. It is perhaps significant that in his youth he was mor-

[1] *Gilles de Rais*, Bossard et Maulde, Paris, 1886.

bidly interested in Seutonius' 'Lives of the Twelve Roman Emperors', with particular emphasis on Caligula, who made a speciality of torturing children.

Peter Kurten, the Dusseldorf murderer, was hanged in 1930, having been found guilty of nine murders and seven attempted murders between February and March 1929. He later confessed to over seventy crimes in the preceding thirty years; of these twenty-two were arson and the rest attacks on men, women and children with hammers, knives, scissors and by manual strangulation. Interviewed by a psychiatrist, Dr Karl Berg,[1] Kurten simply stated that he was impotent unless engaged in extreme violence of this kind. Dr Berg found him intelligent, co-operative and completely without remorse. His childhood was filled with incidents of sexual violence and perversions of all kinds, including those involving animals.

Lesser degrees of sadism are commonplace. Dr Berg himself found a frequent association between early cruelty to animals (often actually encouraged by adults) and later criminality, a trait again exemplified by Ian Brady, the Moors murderer, who used to torture cats as a child.

Stekel[2] says that all cruelty is toned with sexual pleasure. I do not think most people would accept this, not even most psychiatrists, but the combination when evident leads to some of the grossest excesses of individual behaviour known to man.

Masochism

This sexually based enjoyment of pain is not far removed from sadism. It is named after the Austrian novelist, Leopold von Sacher-Masoch (1835–1895), and based on his writings. There are plenty of historical examples of voluntary submission to whipping, notably the religious sect known as the Flagellants, and many of these are thinly disguised sexual perversions. There is of course no disguise

[1] *The Sadist*, Karl Berg, 1938.
[2] *Sadism and Masochism*, Wilhelm Stekel, London, 1955.

about the sort of activity that is purchased every day in the sad world of prostitution; minor degrees of masochism are probably exceedingly common, and the extent to which certain people's evident delight in suffering is a sexual deviation is a matter for serious discussion among psychiatrists. In the course of medical practice one certainly meets a good many patients who are definitely obsessed with their various ills, but most of my colleagues would agree that this on the whole only applies to pain of a comparatively minor degree and embroidered with exaggerations. In the course of thirty years in surgery I have not found anyone who enjoyed really severe pain, though a few patients have refused morphine and allied drugs, preferring pain to clouded mental faculties. There is a pathological craving for pain in certain kinds of idiocy, and self-castration is not uncommon, especially during fits of religious fervour or remorse.

SLAVERY

It is not easy to analyse motives for the more permissive types of cruelty, because infliction of pain is not the prime purpose of the activities leading to it. One common factor is sheer greed, the relentless pursuit of money blinding men to its unfortunate by-products.

Most slaves were regarded as inferior beings, usually easily replaceable, and therefore treated with the utmost callousness, motivated not only by greed but also by any other primitive tendencies their masters (and mistresses) happened to possess. There were exceptions, and in some cases the system worked harmoniously, but never for very long.

Some people imagine that slavery no longer exists, and are astonished to learn that there is an active Anti-Slavery Society today. It recently reported the wholesale use of slaves on rubber plantations in Peru, quelled by whips and dogs and shot if attempting escape; also cases in Syria of children of eight being sold as slaves to private houses. At the time of writing, centres of active slavery are being uncovered in Pakistan and elsewhere, associated with all the ancient conditions of harshness and cruelty.

The practice of slavery ended in the British Dominions in 1811, and in the U.S.A. fifty-four years later. Cuba, with a total population of one and a half million, had 500,000 slaves in 1873, but the children of slaves and the over-sixties were freed, leading to eventual extinction of the system. Brazil abolished slavery in 1883, Ethiopia in 1942. The number of slaves in Arabia is currently estimated as half a million, with mutilations and flogging among the commoner punishments.

The old slave-ships were of course notorious for vile conditions and inhuman treatment; it is one of the illogicalities that make human nature so unpredictable and fascinating that John Newton, who wrote the hymn 'How sweet the Name of Jesus sounds', was previously the master of a slave ship.

CRUELTY TO ANIMALS

The use of animals for food, clothing and research are practical necessities under present conditions; they are therefore considered later. Surely in a different category is the question of amusements at the expense of animals in pain. This seems to be basically wrong, because it is completely unnecessary and cannot fail to induce the kind of callousness that leads easily to persecution on a larger scale.

The spectacle of animals baiting each other or in conflict with men continues to provide highly profitable amusement in many countries and has done so for centuries. The gladiatorial contests in Rome were traditional, and were patronized by the very elect, as are bullfights in Spain today. It is perhaps less well-known that bull-baiting and bear-baiting were extremely popular spectacles in mediaeval England and attracted similar aristocratic patronage, including the reigning monarch. The bears were blinded and tethered to a post with a chain; a bulldog maddened by pain and hunger was then set on the bear, while men with whips stood around and encouraged the animals to fight. Sometimes the bear succeeded in killing the dog before it got too mauled. Queen Elizabeth I was particularly fond of this spectacle.

Cock-fighting is still popular in many countries, including secret sessions in the west and north of England, the animals being fitted with steel claws and fighting to the death. It is a national pastime in Venezuela, watched only by men and boys. Incidentally a fighting cock actually killed the referee in the Philippines in 1961; it is perhaps of interest that the usual English reaction to this information is one of sharp pleasure.

It is not easy to treat *Bullfighting* dispassionately, and I am sometimes told that as I have never seen a bullfight I have no right to venture an opinion on the matter. Most of us have not seen a man on the rack, or a woman burned alive, or a battered baby, or a cat with its tail soaked in petrol and set on fire, but we can hold opinions about such things and say that we would or would not actually wish to witness or indulge in them. Whatever the traditional background to bullfighting, and the skill and courage displayed by the matadors, the cold facts leave no doubt that this intensely commercialized spectacle involves a great deal of pain, because before the animal is killed it is subjected to deliberate injuries to madden and weaken it to the point of complete non-resistance. A few spectators may be upset by the sight of disembowelled horses, but this is a matter of no moment to the *aficionado*. The whole spectacle is decked out with panoply worthy of a gladiator-versus-lion contest in Imperial Rome, and, except that the lion had a rather better chance of winning than the bull, seems to have a very similar appeal.

Hunting for Pleasure

Most hunts involve the pursuit of an individual animal until it is exhausted and terrified, and then its death. The kill often means dragging the creature out of its last futile hiding place and allowing it (for instance) to be torn to pieces by dogs. In many cases, especially in shooting, the animals are bred specially for the sport to ensure an adequate supply. Some kinds of hunting and shooting carry social connotations of a high order and are very expensive to indulge in at the correct level; children brought up in these surroundings are usually sickened by the kill at first, but such softness is soon overcome if taken in hand early enough.

It would be easy to devote a number of pages to the nauseating details that attend the hunting of otters (now almost extinct), hares, foxes and their cubs, as well as the various 'game' birds and many other animals. Two powerful factors help to keep hunting going — the participation of very well-known people, and the support of animal protection societies by wealthy hunting individuals who buy their way into committees and then obstruct legislation against their particular interests.[1]

Arrangements are currently being made in the Hudson Bay area to hunt the rare and harmless white Beluga whale, with harpoons, from speed-boats, for 'sport'. This disgraceful business apparently has the approval of the Premier of Manitoba.

I cannot resist quoting a paragraph by 'Beachcomber' from the *Daily Express*, 22 July 1967:

'Yet another attack on bull-fighting made the amazing admission that a certain degree of courage is shown by the matador. Far greater courage can be seen in this country on any factory farm.

Against overwhelming odds, a daredevil will face the imprisoned pigs and calves, or even a ferocious battery hen. And what of the sportsmen who confront, unflinchingly, untamed hares at a coursing foray? And spare a thought for the intrepid horsemen who, protected only by a few hounds, stand up to a fox at bay.'

A word about performing animals and pets. Few wild animals can be trained without subjection to pain and fear. The ridiculous and degrading tricks that creatures like lions and bears perform in circuses involve months and sometimes years of cruelty that the public never sees and does not want to know about.

The pet trade supplies countless thousands of small animals, birds and fish to shops, fairs and bazaars to be bought or won as prizes, mostly for children and doomed to a short life ended by

[1] For an entirely reasoned, factual and intelligent survey of the subject I strongly recommend *Against Hunting* (A Symposium), edited by Patrick Moore.

neglect, starvation and often cruelty. Millions of guinea pigs, hamsters, tortoises, goldfish and small birds die every year through sheer callousness, having given a few weeks of pleasure. Such a trivial view of living things is bound to have profound psychological effects on those involved.

It is often asserted that an animal's behaviour is instinctive and not the result of thought. One would imagine that this would at least absolve it from criminal responsibility, but in fact there are numerous solemnly recorded examples of the judicial torture and execution of various animals, quite apart from the vast numbers slaughtered in the process of sacrifice to the gods.

In 1266 at Fontenoy-aux-Roses near Paris a pig was burned at the stake for eating a child. In 1386 a sow injured the arms and face of a child; it may be mentioned, I hope without bias, that a sow is unlikely to indulge in such behaviour unless it is being tormented in some way. The tribunal of Falaise sentenced the animal to be 'mangled and maimed in the forelegs and head' and then hanged, and this was duly carried out in the public square, with the wretched creature dressed as a man. In 1394 a pig was hanged for eating a consecrated wafer.

There were plenty of sentences for *bestiality*, the animal being executed with its human partner. A man and a goat were burned alive in Paris for this in 1546, a man and a mule in 1595, and as late as 1726 a man and a mare were burned alive in Germany. These events attracted huge crowds, as did the execution of a cock in 1474 at Basle, for laying an egg. (It was not an egg at all, just some veterinary curiosity.)

Food

Throughout nature one species preys on another for food, and it is easier to justify eating animals than some other activities; indeed if the whole world went vegetarian most of us would die of starvation. It is simple economics that animals in good condition are worth more than those which are not, so on most farms animals destined for food live fairly well. Notable exceptions are the bobby-calves for veal, which are forced into transport for the slaughter-house soon after birth, and the debatable ethics of battery hens and other such animals. The actual slaughter of animals has been the subject of very careful legislation in this country, but even so most people who have visited a slaughter-house find the conditions quite revolting. What legislation there is apparently does not apply to the ritual slaughter of animals for certain religious groups, owing to the necessity for complete exsanguination. This precludes the use of a humane killer or a quick death; the animal is hung up by one leg, or confined upside down in a pen; its throat is cut, and it must then struggle as much as possible to force the blood out of the muscles. In fact the expulsion of every trace of blood from muscles by such means is an impossibility.

Clothing

Certain animals bred in captivity for furs such as mink are on the whole well treated and killed quickly.[1] The vast bulk of furs are taken from animals obtained by trapping, and this is a very different story.

The standard method of catching wild animals for their skins (or as a means of pest control) is a steel spring trap designed to close on a leg and hold it firmly. Careful design is necessary to ensure that the leg is not severed, or so much damaged that the animal is able to tear it away or bite it off. This is accomplished by providing rough teeth, and in the case of large animals like bears, spikes as well to transfix the limb. The power of the jaws snapping closed is frequently enough to break the leg bones, and the skin and muscles are extensively damaged; but of course this is of no consequence to the trapper because the legs are not used in the trade.

The animal's violent efforts to escape obviously result in further damage. Occasionally one does escape, either minus half a leg or with a mangled one, but damaged animals seldom survive long in nature.

How long the animals remain in such traps depends on the men

[1] *Mink on My Shoulder*, R. B. Serjeant.

who visit them. It is found by experience that there is no particular hurry; the pelts do not deteriorate just because of a few days of pain, thirst, hunger and exhaustion, so long as the animal remains alive. Sometimes the helpless creature is attacked and devoured by predators, or it may damage its skin against the ground or other objects in its struggles. This is clearly undesirable, and some clever devices are sometimes used to avoid it; for instance smaller animals can be swung into the air by the trapped limb on a kind of sprung pole. In England the steel trap (gin trap) was not abolished by law until 1958, after years of patient pressure by minorities. It is still used in Scotland.

The annual slaughter of 50,000 baby seals in the Gulf of St. Lawrence was suspended in March 1969 after extensive protests and the publication of pictures like that facing Page 65. One hopes the Canadian Government will not allow this disgraceful business to start again, but the pelts fetch about £30 each.

The number of animals involved in the kind of procedures outlined above is approximately 100 million each year, almost exclusively to provide fur coats for women.

Animal Experiments

No aspect of animal cruelty has caused more outcry than this, under the evocative name Vivisection. Of course hostility on purely emotional grounds is often based on some psychological imbalance, and consequently one witnesses such curious inconsistencies as fox-hunting squires on the committees of animal protection societies, women in furs attending anti-vivisection meetings, a Hampshire clergyman who breeds fighting cocks for export to Peru at £100 each, and a lady member of an anti-vivisection society who shot and maimed a young boy's pet dog because it was chasing her cat.[1]

Let us be perfectly clear on one fundamental point – most medical progress depends on animal experiments. Some anti-vivisectionists say that the results are not applicable to humans. In most cases they are, but in a few it is true that human experiments

[1] *Sunday Express*, 19th March, 1967.

would be more accurate; some of these were conducted by the Nazis on what they regarded as expendable material. Any success achieved in the field of organ transplantation is built on an immense amount of animal research. I am cynical enough to think that an anti-vivisectionist whose child has a potentially fatal heart defect will not refuse the cure offered by modern surgery because it is founded on operativere search using dogs; nor will he forego polio immunization during a scare, knowing that testing the vaccine kills two thousand monkeys every year. An increasing amount of research can be done nowadays with tissue cultures, and this should undoubtedly be done whenever it provides a reasonable alternative to living animals.

The total number of animals used for experimental purposes in England alone now approaches six million a year, mostly cats, dogs, rats, mice and guinea pigs. The vast majority of these experiments do not involve any cutting at all, and hence cannot be called vivi-section, but that some experiments are painful cannot be denied, especially outside England. In England laws governing the use of experimental animals are far more stringent than any protecting pets or the hunted, particularly regarding the infliction of pain. Anybody can torment otters or hares or foxes to death in the name of sport, taking as long as they like about it, but scientists cannot conduct the most trivial experiment on a rat without a licence from the Home Office, regular inspection by fully trained men, and an undertaking to abide by the Pain Rule, which places very definite limits on the amount of suffering that may be caused. An anaesthetic must be given for any procedure involving more pain than a simple injection, and if subsequent suffering is likely the animal must be painlessly killed. Undoubtedly these regulations are not always observed, but outside England little or no protection exists and innumerable experiments of extreme cruelty are done. Sir Joseph Barcroft, the eminent British physiologist, had to leave a French laboratory because 'the cruelty going on there was going to make him vomit'.

We can in fact easily produce facts to show that the English strongly lead the world in legislation for animal protection, but there is nothing whatever in our history to show that we naturally possess such a tendency. Most of this legislation has been very recent and introduced only after repeated and forceful action by vociferous minorities. In England before this happened, and at the present time in most of the rest of the world, cruelty to animals or indifference to their sufferings can only be described as commonplace.

So far as our love for animals is concerned the short answer is that we love certain specified nice-looking well-behaved creatures: horses (for riding), doggies, pussies, robins, budgies and most baby animals. Our attitude towards animals like rabbits, guinea pigs, foxes and deer is ambivalent, a highly esteemed term stolen from chemistry by the psychoanalysts and meaning (in this context) that we can love them or not depending on how we feel. The rat, an intelligent and sensitive creature, is regarded with unequivocal fear and hatred; so are snakes and spiders. Animals in other countries are not really our concern; although we may disapprove of our friends' behaviour it is not done to criticize openly.

The RSPCA

In England the Royal Society for the Prevention of Cruelty to Animals was founded in 1824, and it is the oldest of all animal protection societies. It now has an invested capital of £2,500,000 (the National Society for the Prevention of Cruelty to Children has £924,000), and maintains about two hundred inspectors in this country alone. The Society very rightly lays great theoretical stress on juvenile education in relation to animal cruelty, but has no real power in this vital matter and takes a singularly negative attitude in the subject of fox-hunting. It has been responsible for vast improvements in the iniquitous treatment of animals for food and for 'pets', as well as in trapping for pest control. The Society's efforts in regard to legislation for the protection of performing animals and for those submitted to ritual slaughter have been defeated in both Houses of Parliament several times.

Some may feel that too much space has been devoted to animal cruelty, but there are several reasons for this emphasis; the first of these is simply to call attention to some unpleasant facts. The amount of pain that is deliberately inflicted on animals, or that they are allowed to suffer, is beyond all calculation. The outline here is in fact pitifully inadequate, but it does attempt to give a glimpse of activities to which many quite kindly people just shut their minds. The second reason is to underline the dual nature of this matter – we are concerned not only with the animals' pain but also with the effects of such cruelty on the people concerned, especially children. These effects are far deeper and more powerful than might be expected, and there are innumerable examples (apart from the two I have quoted) of murderers and sadists whose childhood was warped in this way. The relevance of these things is not to be measured by their place in time. Bear-baiting was abolished many years ago; not, it has been said, because it gave pain to the bear but because it gave pleasure to the spectators. Bullfighting continues today; yet it was condemned in 1567, when the Inquisition was still active, by a Papal Bull (!) in these words: 'It is sinful to torture dumb animals. Such sins are degrading to the soul and disposition of the tormentor.'

The third reason is that animal cruelty exemplifies an attitude towards pain that touches basic and menacing characteristics in our nature, and these may need enormous efforts to eradicate if we are to survive as a species; this aspect will be referred to again at the end of the book.

ENDURANCE

The full reasons and motives behind extremes of endurance are really unfathomable, but we can think about the more obvious ones. Making every allowance for bias, exaggeration, wishful thinking and propaganda, it does seem beyond doubt that a few men and women have endured the very worst pain that ingenious and ruthless people could devise rather than renounce their faith, show cowardice, or betray their friends. Such conduct is extremely rare. In the dungeons of the Inquisition confessions of heresy or witchcraft meant death at the stake, yet failure to obtain confession was very exceptional. There are various accounts of people being burned alive and 'bearing their sufferings with fortitude, in steadfast silence'. One finds it difficult to credit this, and most eye-witness reports unbiased by religious fervour describe the victims writhing and screaming once reached by the flames, including Joan of Arc, whose 'shrieks and lamentations moved several to pity'.[1]

Yet the few cannot be broken – why?

The main component seems to be the sheer strength of *belief* in something – in the absolute rightness of one's religion, in reward for tenacity or punishment for giving way, in the impossibility of living with a betrayal on one's conscience, even in one's own power of defiance. In 1665 Dr Elscholtz operated on an Army officer for a perineal tumour; he refused to be tied down because 'it was not becoming to a soldier'. Many recorded cases have been in connection with various religions – men tortured and dying painfully for their faith without yielding. The vital point is not whether these beliefs are true or false – they cannot all be true – but men's intensity of faith in them, which can be complete.

Another factor is a curious inborn quality of *stubbornness*, observable even in quite small babies when they don't want to do something required of them. It turns up in the most unexpected people, sometimes apparently feeble and ineffective, who cling to some trivial possession or opinion in the face of all reason, or to a belief against any tyranny.

Threshold and *tolerance* have already been mentioned, and undoubtedly some people feel pain less than others. The complexity of the pathways inevitably means differences, and probably this can be considerable, even at extremes.

A severe pain can be acceptable or resented, depending mainly on the reason for its infliction. A number of people can steel themselves to very severe pain if they know that what is being done to them is the only possible way out of a desperate situation and that it is being carried out as rapidly and efficiently as possible. This applies occasionally even today, but did so much more in connection with surgical procedures before anaesthesia. Perhaps a similar process obtained in the exaltation of martyrdom, where the *certainty* of ineffable glory might reduce mere physical pain to an insignificant level, especially perhaps if death was inevitable, as in crucifixion and the stake.

The actual *method* of producing pain must have some bearing on the matter, not because some procedures are more painful than

[1] *Superstition and Force*, H. C. Lea.

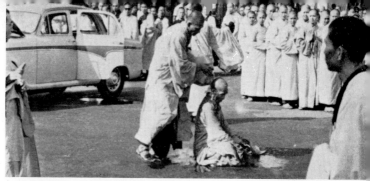
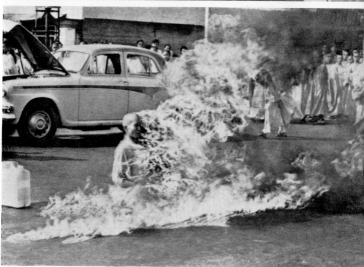
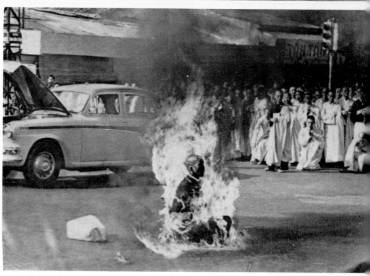

3 Buddhist monk voluntarily drenched in petrol and burned alive. Saigon 1963. (See p. 97) *Photo: Associated Press*

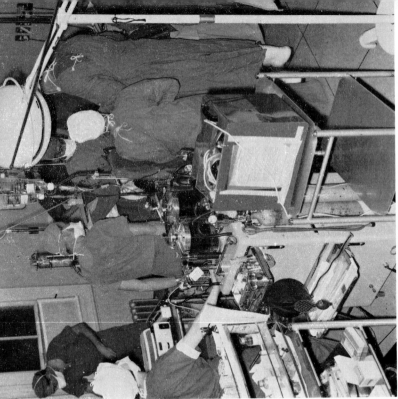

4b The complexity of modern anaesthesia is exemplified by this picture of a patient undergoing heart surgery. (See p. 130)

Photo: R. Leng

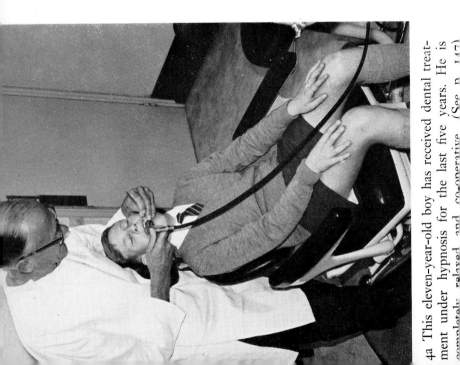

4a This eleven-year-old boy has received dental treatment under hypnosis for the last five years. He is completely relaxed and co-operative. (See p. 147)

others, but because of their special significance to certain people. It is probably true to say that there is an upper limit to the pain that can be experienced by any particular individual, so that the psyche can be saturated by crushing a single finger, and the total amount of pain would not be increased by simultaneously crushing another finger, or all of them. But people may find some things more intolerable than pain, having perhaps an unquenchable horror of blindness or some other mutilation. Tearing out people's nails produces about as much pain as anything else one can do, but it does not result in much permanent disability and is not an intrinsically degrading process. A very few people are in any case untorturable, because they faint every time the slightest thing is done.

We do not have to look back very far to find examples of people voluntarily submitting to extremes of pain for some special cause. The Buddhist monks and nuns in Vietnam who voluntarily burned themselves to death with petrol apparently sustained this process with serenity.

I am not a Buddhist monk and I do not have synthetic beliefs powerful enough to modify the pain of a sprained ankle, let alone burning alive. If I were selected for such a purpose, I should expect my colleagues to support my gesture to the extent of ensuring that it would not fail, and as far as I am concerned this would mean providing me with a capsule of potassium cyanide that I could bite as soon as the petrol was ignited. This would kill me in a matter of seconds, and since a post-mortem would not be performed there would be no risk of detection. I am not denying that modifying impulses can be generated voluntarily in the higher centres to the extent of cancelling the reactions to pain, if not pain itself; only that no normal person can do this. Quite major operations can be done painlessly under hypnosis, and hysterical phenomena include completely painless major injuries and burns; all these presumably lead to blocks generated in the higher centres by purely mental activities, and there is no scientific reason why similar processes should not be generated as the result of an effort of will. Intense mental training (such as that in esoteric Buddhism) supplemented by intense desire, may result in this power.

There are numerous records of bizarre suicides by people who in former days would have been called 'mad'. One man drove a red-hot crow-bar into his abdomen; another hammered a ten-inch cold-chisel completely through his head from side to side, followed by another from the front which reached a depth of four inches before he died. Such feats are completely impossible unless the mind is profoundly disturbed, and it seems likely that in this respect the mental processes behind madness and martyrdom are not very different.

Certain prisoners in Nazi concentration camps subjected to repeated beatings and other abuses over long periods became almost accustomed to them. Leon Wells[1] says, 'It is said that people get hardened to pain. I believe from my experience that this is so. Without realizing it one begins to apply what is called *self-hypnotism* to shut off certain connections between the brain and the body.' He goes on to say that the pain from beatings consciously diminished, but that *hunger* was felt to be the greatest pain, and they would sustain twenty-five lashes for a bit of bread.

The patient endurance of long-continued pain of a more chronic type without complaint is almost as remarkable – in some ways more so. Many victims of arthritis and other sources of unceasing pain keep their suffering very much to themselves, mainly perhaps because the average healthy person has very little capacity for sympathy lasting more than a few minutes, after which the matter becomes boring. Thus pain, the weariness, the insomnia and the periodic despair are kept secret for as long as possible, in a few cases with help from an understanding doctor. The fortitude displayed by some of these people is almost beyond belief; in my experience it has little connection with religion.

PENALTIES

EQUIPPED as we are with all these potentialities for cruelty and violence it is hardly surprising that we indulge in individual or group acts of this kind when in anger, or even that mass persecution of hated or feared minorities should break out from time to time.

[1] *The Janowska Road*, Leon Wells.

One would not perhaps expect things to go much further than this, but the grim reality is that the infliction of pain has always been, and still is, an integral part of legal systems all over the world.

But surely we are much more enlightened and refined than we used to be; what purpose therefore can there be in reviewing these sordid details from history? Regretfully one must face the fact that any improvement is illusory, depending far more on a temporary high standard of living for the masses than on any genetic developments. Modifications of attitude have also resulted from the vast improvement in communications, the establishment of democracies, some of the scientific advances, universal education, comparatively unbiased judical systems, and the decline of religious autocracy. If these and other standards are departed from, entire nations can revert to pure savagery in the name of Law, and unless they are then brought under control the world could once again be dominated by conditions closely resembling those of the ancient world and of the Middle Ages; a brief review of some of these conditions is therefore doubly relevant in a book about pain, bearing in mind that we are genetically and indeed intellectually hardly different from the people concerned — also that practically all the varieties of cruelty mentioned were applied on a huge scale during both World Wars, and that more are continually being disclosed.

So far as the actual methods of inflicting pain are concerned any detailed account would be out of place here, but a few examples call for comment. In general the methods are related to the known sensitivity of the skin and other parts of the body as outlined in Part I, and much ingenuity has been used in devising some of them. Their efficacy, however, is due more to the circumstances and to the individuals concerned, and a man is as likely to be rendered compliant or insane by the use of a box of matches as by all the armamentarium in the dungeons of the Inquisition.

Flogging is by far the commonest form of punishment by pain, mainly because it is so easy. Although plenty of people have been beaten to death the general idea seems to be the production of pain without vital loss or impairment, the victim being intended to survive with revised viewpoints. Oddly enough beatings and whippings have never been regarded as forms of torture unless inflicted in some unusual site, such as the soles of the feet (bastinado).

The administration of a beating seems to be almost instinctive as a means of correction or retribution or punishment. Even the most gentle and compassionate of people are sometimes goaded into action of this kind, especially if matters of principle are involved:

And when he had made a scourge of small cords, he drove them all out of the temple, and the sheep, and the oxen; and poured out the changers' money, and overthrew the tables.

(St John II, 15)

The application of *heat* in various forms has always been favoured as an effective means of causing legal pain. The methods include naked flames, roasting, and searing or scalding the skin with hot objects such as irons or stones and with water or oil or molten lead. These procedures are of great antiquity and almost universal in distribution.

The various kinds of punitive *mutilation* practised widely by savage tribes and by 'civilized' people when given the opportunity mainly entailed alterations to the visible skin surfaces, notably the face. In India the usual punishment for adultery was to cut off a man's nose (presumably to render him less attractive) and this led to some very ingenious plastic surgery — identical in many ways with modern rhinoplasty — notably by a highly skilled Indian surgeon named Susutra in the fifth century AD. The operations involve transference of skin from other parts of the body and the use of pedicle skin-flaps from the forehead. It will be appreciated that no anaesthetics were available.

Many savage tribes practice mutilation of the skin in the course of initiation and other ceremonies of a religious nature; some of the procedures must have been extremely painful, but no man or boy dared show any sign of it for fear of disgrace. However in many cases alcohol or a kind of hypnosis resulted in at least partial anaesthesia. In England the tyrannical Forest Laws beginning with Canute in 1016 resulted in wholesale lopping off of hands and other features for poaching. Under Henry I, coiners who escaped capital punishment lost at least one hand and often their testicles as well. Quite recently King Feisal of Saudi Arabia is quoted as saying that the penalty of cutting off a man's hand for theft is still carried out; he added 'There is very little crime in my country'.

The acute tenderness of the *nail-beds* has received much attention from specialists in inflicting pain, and particularly favoured by modern practitioners. It does seem extraordinary that anyone could stand having all their toenails avulsed, with the prospect of ten further episodes on their fingers, yet this has apparently been achieved.[1]

SPECIAL DEVICES

The *rack* was probably the most common instrument of all in use throughout the ancient world and Mediaeval Europe. Most gaolers soon discovered that a second session after a day or two was more effective because of the greatly increased sensitivity (hyperalgesia) of the damaged joints. Dislocations were common; the more expert operators would reduce these for the richer clients when the procedure was over.

The rack was used for day after day on Guy Fawkes (1570–1606) eventually forcing him to disclose the names of his accomplices and sign a confession. It is an interesting sidelight on the times that the official edict authorizing his torture (signed by King James I) directed that 'the gentler tortures should be used first'. So far as one can tell this would entail suspending him by his thumbs – a mere trifle.

The *Torture Chair* in Horniman's Museum, South East London, is equipped with numerous mechanical devices of horrible ingenuity. This beautifully made example of the blacksmith's art was discovered in a dungeon used by the Inquisition in Quenca. It was made in 1676, and bought by a Mr Willett in 1898 for £200, to be exhibited in Brighton. The original notice read: 'This awful instrument is exhibited to remind the Visitor of the danger of our being conceited enough to wish to Compel others to think like ourselves – the foundations of Bigotry and Persecution.'

Crucifixion is regarded as a special case because it was used for the execution of Christ. It was in fact used freely in Roman law at

[1] *Odette*, Gerard Tickell.

the time, invariably preceded by flogging. It was very common in the ancient world, especially favoured by the Phoenicians and Carthaginians; in 519 BC Darius of Persia crucified three thousand political prisoners in Babylon.

It is a remarkably cruel way of killing people, combining skin, muscle, nerve, joint and bone damage with the adjuncts of exposure, thirst, humiliation and asphyxia. Modern research shows that the crucified man could only breathe by taking the weight off his arms, and after his legs were broken he soon died, so this was in fact an act of mercy. Nearly all pictures and statues of formal crucifixions are anatomically and physiologically impossible. Nails through the palms could not be used to suspend a man – they would tear out between the fingers. The nails were driven through the wrists, as shown in Langhetti's painting, and in this position transfixed the median (sensory) nerve. There are plenty of modern instances of crucifixion, particularly during the World Wars.

LEGALIZED CRUELTY

History is replete with accounts of organized and legalized cruelty in the form of torture and barbaric capital punishments, extending over thousands of years in the whole of the civilized world.

It must be remembered that the development of a satisfactory and just legal system is no easy matter. To punish criminals and petty offenders is easy enough, so long as there has been a definite offence and the culprit is found; his punishment is then usually automatic. Although by present New World standards it may seem fantastically stupid and cruel to cut off a man's hand for stealing a shilling or two, undoubtedly harsh penalties were once necessary, and they were well known to the potential criminal. At all times the real difficulty has been to find the criminal and then to prove his guilt; when this is combined with expendable masses, feudal systems, religious intolerance, slavery and god-like dictatorships, cruelty becomes inevitable. Even so a few civilizations kept it to a minimum, legally at any rate. There are very few references to torture being used legally to obtain evidence in ancient Egypt (though one of these dates from about 1200 BC in the reign of Rameses XI), and torture has never been legal in English Common Law.

One of the oldest systems in the world for apportioning responsibility was the *ordeal*. Where it proved impossible, because of conflicting evidence, or the complete lack of it, to be certain of a person's guilt or to decide between several possibilities the ordeal was held to be the final proof. It consisted in making the suspect take some action that would normally cause violent pain, probably severe injury and possibly death. If he came through this unscathed he was held to be innocent and released; if not he was guilty and suffered accordingly. That a very satisfactory number of convictions was secured can be inferred from the nature of the procedures used. These included carrying red-hot iron in the hands, walking barefoot on red-hot ploughshares, licking red-hot axes, fishing stones out of cauldrons of boiling water or oil, taking poisons and powerful emetics, and being bitten by venomous snakes. All these devices had been (and still are) used by primitive tribes, and they persisted with little change well into the twelfth and thirteenth centuries as part of Western law.

The tests of the ordeal died hard, in spite of condemnation by Pope Innocent III in 1215. The ordeal by red-hot iron was used all over Europe until at least 1500; Lea[1] says that ordeal by boiling oil was recorded in a case of theft at Benares in 1783, and another unofficial one was described in the *Bombay Gazette* in 1867.

If divine intervention were the deciding factor it seems curious that the simple and humane method of casting lots was not more popular as a means of settling disputes. This of course was not in the least spectacular (and hence unremunerative) so it was condemned by Pope Leo VI as 'mere divination'. Perhaps more important was the fact that it was not painful, and so failed to satisfy certain primitive appetites.

Judicial Torture

There never had been a time when torture was not legal in certain

[1] *Superstition and Force*, H. C. Lea.

circumstances, so it was freely employed, notably for the underdog in systems of slavery and feudalism; there was no practical limit to what a master could do to his slaves or a lord to his villeins and serfs. Any history of such systems shows a plenitude of floggings, torture, burnings or mutilations for the smallest offences. However, although these practices were condoned or overlooked by the laws of the country, that is not at all the same thing as the deliberate use of torture judicially in civilized communities; this occurred to a vast extent over hundreds of years in the ancient world, and again in the Middle Ages in Europe. In fact, Lea says, 'Torture has received the sanction of the wisest law-givers during the greater part of the world's history'.[1]

In the earliest Greek and Roman law torture was used mainly on slaves, but these constituted most of the working population of the countries, including teachers and other professions. The total population of Rome in the first century AD was about one and a half million, of whom, according to Josephus, one million were slaves. Its legal system was by far the most highly developed in the world at the time.

Under Roman law a slave's evidence was not accepted as proof unless obtained under torture, so it was freely applied in most civil cases requiring evidence. Roman law did however embody certain restrictions on the use of torture, and in theory these gave some protection. It was only allowed to be used after formal accusation, and if this was found to be without foundation the accuser was himself liable to be tortured. It was definitely illegal to torture anyone after confession to implicate others, in marked contrast to later developments. Torture was not used on women during pregnancy or on children under fourteen, and it was only supposed to be used after all other means had been tried and final proof was necessary. It was restricted to slaves except in cases of *majestas* (*lèse-majesté*) or treason, when there were few restrictions of rank or sex or age. Later on even these restrictions became farcical, and when fear for the constitution was at its height a man of high rank was tortured on suspicion of *majestas* because he carried a coin with the Emperor's image on it into a public lavatory.

[1] H. C. Lea, *op. cit.*

At this time many eminent Romans strongly condemned torture as a means of getting evidence – not so much on humanitarian grounds as because such evidence was unreliable; a tough guilty man might resist almost anything, while the weaker innocent one would falsely confess to avoid further torment. Among writers against torture were Adrian, Cicero, and Quintilian (AD 35–95) who also condemned corporal punishment of children.

The Romans were basically tough aggressive peasants, and their 'culture' was like a Stradivarius varnish on a rotting oak plank. When they had no worlds left to conquer they turned their intrinsic cruelty towards their slaves and criminals, and eventually on themselves, thus achieving their own destruction. Compared, however, with subsequent Christian activities their behaviour was moderate and restrained.

There is much to support the belief that ancient Greece was the ideal civilization, combining unequalled culture with the worship of all that was fine and beautiful, including the human body. While Romans gloated over public spectacles of men being tortured to death, Greeks listened to Sophocles and watched naked athletes under the Athenian sun. But defence against aggressors was a constant need, as was punishment of criminals; moreover slavery was part of the system, as was the use of eunuchs and hence professional castrators. We also find torture by standard methods as part of the Greek judicial system, though on nothing like the Roman scale. Sadism and masochism were rare, probably because of the almost complete sexual freedom; the only sexual crimes were those against children before puberty and those featuring violence.

The Spartans had the reputation of ruthless harshness, a necessity imposed by their position as a minority at great risk. Plutarch tells us that deformed or feeble children were exposed by law in a gorge on Mount Taygetus. Boys were taken from their mothers at the age of seven and brought up in the strictest discipline, with floggings for punishment and as a test of endurance.

Greek morality was based on punishment for crime, for offences against the state, and for acts that were unjust to others. Intolerance was relatively rare, in spite of a religious system of unprecedented and unequalled complexity – or perhaps because of this; most Greeks must have regarded the gods and their activities with almost benevolent amusement and pride.

After the fall of the Roman Empire there was no great centre of civilization west of Constantinople for hundreds of years; with an uneasy truce between Church and State torture ceased to be a prominent part of judicial systems, though having periodical exacerbations. Its use was strongly opposed by St Augustine and by Gregory I in the sixth century AD, and by Nicholas I in the ninth century. During this period doubtful cases were often tried by ordeal and by the curious custom known as the Wager of Battle, where the two sides were required to fight it out personally (or with assigned 'Champions') in the form of a duel. This was undoubtedly another discouragement to frivolous litigation, especially as the loser, if not killed in the duel, was likely to be hanged or very heavily fined.

In England the development of the feudal system brought innumerable centres of oppression and cruelty, every castle having its dungeons and assortment of do-it-yourself torture instruments. Occasionally outbursts of savagery occurred on a national scale, depending largely on the temperament of the current monarch and the state of his coffers. In 1210 King John had a great round-up of Jews all over England and forced them by imprisonment and torture to pay enormous ransoms.

The Holy Church

Conditions like this prevailed over most of the civilized world until the early thirteenth century, with short shrift for the poor, the petty offender, vagrants and dissenters, but torture not forming any definite part of the law. However, as the Church gained power in Europe it also grew intolerant and began to interest itself to a much greater extent in the one activity that could undermine its domination – heresy. The extent to which the Church ultimately possessed not only the bodies and minds of men but the State as well may seem inconceivable until we remember quite similar domination by the Nazi régime in recent years.

At the beginning of the thirteenth century the Roman Catholic Church, through Pope Innocent III, began to sharpen its claws, and from that time on the Inquisition system grew in strength all over the Continent, although there was no fixed central policy except the invariable and profitable one of confiscating all the victims' property for the Holy Church. Burning heretics at the stake first became statutory law in Aragon in 1197; the practice spread, and by the middle of the thirteenth century was the standard method of execution. As always, biblical justification was found, in John xv, 6: '*If a man abide not in me, he is cast forth as a branch, and is withered; and men gather them, and cast them unto the fire, and they are burned.*'

The Inquisition not only interpreted this as an instruction to burn people who did not conform with its particular tenets, but also to burn them alive and fully conscious.

There were then few obstacles to absolute power. One was that 'free confession' was necessary, and it is not very hard to guess how this problem was solved. In 1252 Pope Innocent IV issued instructions to the Inquisition at Lombardy and Tuscany that torture was to be used on all suspected heretics to obtain confessions, and after that they were to be tortured further to force them to name accomplices.

The unending flow of confessed heretics obtained by this chain-reaction method can be easily imagined, each bringing revenue to the Church in the form of confiscated possessions. No one was exempt, and the richer the victim the bigger the prize. Only one handicap remained.

It was an essential part of Church dogma at the time that no ecclesiastic should be a direct party to bloodshed or death; arguments that the rack and the strappado did not actually draw blood were felt to be questionable, so the torture and execution of victims had been placed in the hands of secular authoriües. This was a considerable disadvantage, and the final iniquity was a Papal Bull of 1256 allowing absolution to priests concerned in the torture of suspects. Thus the system became completely secret within the Church, with no possibility of defence, appeal, or escape. The alleged heretics were hunted like rats and shown less mercy. Execution by burning at the *Auto-da-Fé* was left to the secular authorities, but conducted as a public spectacle with full Church panoply and ritual.

The hold of the Church over entire countries from the monarch down was complete. Any man taking high office had to swear that he would prosecute heresy with zeal, or risk excommunication or worse. And this state of affairs lasted for over four hundred years.

Truly, '*It is a fearful thing to fall into the hands of the living God.*' (Hebrews x, 31.)

It is hardly surprising that the civil authorities in Europe, with the full blessing of the Church, adopted much the same principles into a system already redolent with cruelty. Suspects were being tortured for evidence and for the names of accomplices with great regularity, and the practice became incorporated into judicial systems with the full approval of eminent legal authorities, leading to exactly the same abuses and excesses as were current in the Inquisition.

The first official reference to the use of judicial torture in Europe comes from Amiens in 1283. By 1380 it was freely employed even for trivial cases all over France, without even the slender safeguards of the Roman system. As an illustration of the conditions obtaining at this time and for the next three hundred years, a single case will suffice, quoted by H. C. Lea[1] from official records in Paris:

> 'A certain Fleurant de Saint-Leu was accused of stealing a silver buckle on January 4th, 1390. He denied it and was tortured twice; he then confessed, but pleaded that it was his first offence. On January 8th the court decided that as the offence was not sufficient to merit death they would find one that was, and he was tortured three times but without success. On the 13th he was again tortured twice, and then admitted that three years previously he had married a prostitute in Senlis. He was kept in a dungeon for three months, and as nothing further was found when the court again discussed his case on April 9th he was hanged the same day.'

[1] *Superstition and Force*, H. C. Lea.

Sorcery and Witchcraft

In England and Europe these were not taken very seriously until the fourteenth century; in fact the Church at first tended to discourage belief in such evident nonsense. However when the Inquisition got really established it started fierce persecution of any activity of this kind as the worst form of heresy, since a pact with the devil was implicit. It therefore fomented belief in all the puerile and fictitious structure of witchcraft, extorting confessions by torture and burning the victims at the stake. England was much slower to adopt this attitude, and even at the height of the witch scare records show that Justices in many cases attempted fair trial and even found some of the accused innocent. The total number of death sentences for witchcraft by hanging or burning in England between 1542 and 1735 was less than a thousand, according to a very careful historian.[1]

Nevertheless witch-hunting became a mania and at its worst involved gross cruelty. The accepted methods of detecting a witch were to throw her into a pond (if she floated she was guilty); to keep her awake by any convenient painful method for anything up to three days; and to find the 'witches' spots' already mentioned, these insensitive areas being craftily hidden by Satan and accordingly requiring skilled and prolonged search. All this led to the profession of 'witch-finder'; these men, at one time headed by the notorious Matthew Hopkins, were paid by results and were responsible for many innocent people being tortured, hanged and burned alive.

The persecution of witches was much more severe in Scotland, where frank torture to secure confessions was usual and burnings frequent. Judicial torture for this or any other purpose was officially abolished there in 1709, but it certainly continued to be used long after that. All this hardly compares with the insensate fury of persecution by the Inquisition, which burned witches (including young children) in hundreds at a time; the Bishop of Wurzburg is said to have burned nine hundred in three months. The total number can only be guessed, but an official record states that thirty thousand were burned between 1404 and 1554, and the true figure is certainly vastly greater.

[1] *A Mirror of Witchcraft*, Christina Hole.

In 1408 in France the number of applications of torture was limited to three, and at the same time the Council of Rheims forbade torturing prisoners to death on feast days – that would be sacrilege, they said.

Other countries, including Germany, were slower to adopt torture judicially but they all did eventually to some degree. The first reference to it in Hungary was in 1514 and by this time it was almost universal elsewhere. Its use was absolutely at the discretion of the judge, who usually had to attend its application; it was decidedly in the judge's interest to secure a confession and one does not imagine leniency was evident. Most countries laid down that 'torture should not be so severe or prolonged as to endanger the patient [sic] permanently'. But this provision was completely farcical in practice, and von Boden, writing in 1600, says: 'Human ingenuity could not invent suffering more terrible than is constantly and legally employed, and Satan himself would be unable to increase its refinements.'

As in the Ancient World the worst of all civil crimes was lèse-majesté, and an actual attempt on a King's life was the ultimate in this category, calling for retribution of the severest kind that could be devised. The attempted assassination of Louis XV in 1757 by Robert François Damiens resulted in one of the most hideous legal sentences in history. There was of course no doubt about the man's guilt, but after his trial he was tortured for two hours with the Boot in an unsuccessful attempt to secure the names of accomplices, until his legs were crushed to pulp. He was then taken to the Place de Gréve in Paris and the precisely detailed sentence of the court carried out in front of a huge crowd. It included burning off his right hand holding the dagger, the application of red-hot pincers to most of his body, and filling the wounds with molten lead, boiling oil and flaming sulphur. This took several hours. One of the executioners found the work distasteful and paid a servant a hundred louis to do it for him. Damiens was then pulled to pieces by four horses, a process that apparently also took over an hour. Among the crowd watching this performance was Casanova, who confessed that it upset him.

Anyone who has inspected the dungeons and their equipment in the Tower of London would at once conclude that the English were as bad as anyone else in the matter of judicial cruelty, and so far as details were concerned this is undoubtedly true; but in fact torture was never part of the English Common Law, even in the Middle Ages. This did mean that ordinary people in ordinary courts could not be legally tortured to obtain either evidence or confessions, or to implicate others; but in exceptional cases, especially those involving sedition or treason, permission was obtainable from the Crown or indeed from any higher court. There are numerous examples of documents permitting torture signed by the reigning monarch, including the terrible Royal Warrant regarding the English Templars in 1310, signed by Edward II at the 'request' of Pope Clement V. Using imported Inquisitors, confessions of unnatural vice, spitting on the cross and other absurdities were wrung out of all but three Templars in the whole of England, and their elimination followed.

Although torture was not permitted under English Common Law there were plenty of ways round this. Flogging did not count as torture, neither did the vile prison conditions. One handicap to litigation was a simple refusal to plead, and various devices were used to force the reluctant prisoner to do so. One of these known as '*peine forte et dure*' consisted in placing a board over the victim and piling weights on it until he consented to plead. This was not counted as torture either, and it was not abolished until 1772, although torture of political prisoners ceased officially in 1640.

There was no restriction on cruelty in *punishment*, and as confession was not necessary a conviction was easy enough, especially in the case of people now known as under-privileged.

Branding was frequently ordered, usually to mark a man for life on the face or hands. The sentence was often carried out in open court. It was abolished from our law in 1829.

Whipping was the commonest of all sentences, and in the sixteenth century ordinary vagrants were whipped naked tied to the back of a cart, a method specifically sanctioned by the Whipping Act of 1530; the executioner was paid 4d a time. Two hundred years later the statutory sentence was slightly modified; the victim was only stripped to the waist and tied to a special whipping post instead of a cart. Every village in England had its own whipping post and a great many of these still stand; a place without one only officially counted as a hamlet.

Corporal punishment existed from very early times in the British Army and Navy, and was often inflicted barbarously on slight occasion. At the beginning of the nineteenth century sentences of 1,000 lashes were common for mutiny and other offences, even in peace time. The cat-o'-nine-tails was 'suspended' (not abolished) from naval law in 1881.

Under English Law in 1967 corporal punishment (which means the 'cat' and the birch) could still be legally awarded in male prisons, for mutiny, encitement to mutiny, and gross personal violence to a prison officer. It could only be ordered by a visiting committee which included at least two justices of the peace, and the order had to be confirmed by the Secretary of State. The Home Secretary refused to confirm such an order following disturbances in Maidstone Gaol in 1967, and corporal punishment in prisons was completely abolished from our law by Section 65 of the Criminal Justice Act, 1967.

Capital Punishment in the Middle Ages was usually by hanging – the slow strangulation kind – performed in public. It was awarded for quite trivial offences and the records include children hanged for stealing a few pence. Under Henry VIII, 72,000 people were hanged in thirty-seven years. Stealing more than one shilling was punishable by death in England until 1808. There was a public hanging in Northampton in 1852, of one Elizabeth Pinckhard, for murder. The last in England was Michael Barrett, for causing the Fenian explosion in Clerkenwell; he was publicly hanged outside Newgate Prison on May 26th 1868. My grandfather was forty at the time, but did not attend. The last official public execution in Europe was that of Eugen Weidman, who was guillotined for murder on June 17th 1939, in Versailles. Elsewhere in the world various Governments temporarily in power conduct such activities with unabated energy.

Burning alive was common in Anglo-Saxon times later for heretics. The first officially recorded victim in England was Alban in 304, and the last was Christian Murphy, who was burned alive for coining on March 18th 1789. The sentence of burning alive was used with great enthusiasm by Mary (1553–1558) when she restored the Roman Catholic religion in England. At least three hundred people died at the stake, including the Prebendary of St Paul's, the Bishop of Gloucester, Ridley and Latimer, and Cranmer.

Henry VIII revived the ancient punishment of *boiling to death* for poisoners in 1531; two men were so executed publicly in King's Lynn and one in Smithfield in the same year. The Act was repealed by Edward VI in 1547.

There is no *official* record of judical torture being used in England after 1640, though as we have seen this is decidedly misleading. Jardine,[1] writing in 1837, points out that since it was never part of our law, 'it is not expressly forbidden by Act of Parliament'.

Torture was officially abolished in Austria in 1780, Saxony 1783, in Russia (by Imperial Ukas) in 1801, and in the Duchy of Baden in 1831.

Although officially abolished in France in 1789 it continued in an emasculated Inquisition and elsewhere for nearly another hundred years, and cases of judicial torture were reported in Prussia and Spain as late as 1879.

CRUELTY TO CHILDREN

The grim history of warfare and persecution includes innumerable examples of children being assaulted and murdered. A good deal of this has been done for the express purpose of hurting the adult population as much as possible, so we find cases of children being tortured in front of their helpless parents, and other atrocities. Mob violence during invasion and suppression of minorities frequently includes the rape of all females, even the youngest children.

In the English Industrial Revolution children up to ten years old (in some cases as young as four) were compelled before 1842 to work in mills and factories under appalling conditions, ill-fed, ill-clothed, beaten frequently and dying in hundreds of neglect and disease. In 1878 the law was amended to allow a twelve-hour day at the age of twelve. A little earlier boys between six and ten years old were used by chimney sweeps — the notorious 'climbing-boys'. These wretched children were usually purchased by their masters, who then had

[1] *On the Use of Torture in the Criminal Law of England*, David Jardine.

absolute power over them; an agile six-year-old might be worth eight pounds, but at nine they were too big and worth only ten shillings or so. The chimney passages were often as small as nine inches square with right-angle bends, and the children had to struggle along these, usually naked. Failure to progress was often interpreted as defiance, and sometimes a fire was lighted to force them on. They worked an average of fifteen hours a day and many died in the process. Protests against this iniquitous system were little heeded; they were led by Jonas Hanway in 1760 (please look carefully at these dates). Action started in Parliament in 1788 and the practice was finally made illegal in 1840. However it went on until sweeps were licensed in 1875. The prevalence of drunkenness at this period did nothing to help these children.

In England there was no legal protection for ill-treated children until 1882, when the Liverpool Society for the Prevention of Cruelty to Children was started by the Reverend Benjamin Waugh, and it succeeded in guiding legislation, reporting cases of cruelty and helping parents where this was indicated. Since 1884 the National Society for Prevention of Cruelty to Children has dealt with approximately three million cases. The total number in 1965–1966 was 39,929 – well over a hundred a day. This, of course, represents only a minute fraction of what actually occurs, mainly because people are too cowardly or stupid to report what they frequently see happening. It is not the policy of the Society to prosecute if this can possibly be avoided and less than a thousand cases reached the courts in 1965–1966.

It should be mentioned that anyway penalties for extreme cruelty to children are not severe. Wilful assault causing 'unnecessary suffering or injury to health, including injury to or loss of sight, or limb or organ of the body, or any emotional derangement' is only a misdemeanour, and the maximum penalty on conviction in a magistrates' court is six months imprisonment and/or a fine of twenty-five pounds. (The maximum penalty for cruelty to an animal is exactly double this.) If the case goes for trial, conviction can still only result in two years imprisonment and/or a fine of one hundred pounds. In a recent case a child was blinded for life and probably sustained permanent brain damage after being repeatedly punched in the face by his father. The man was fined twenty-five pounds – probably a week's wages. The prevalence of callous violence to children has even resulted in a new medical category – the 'battered baby' syndrome; it includes multiple fractures of the skull and of the limbs. These cases are undoubtedly increasing in frequency, to such an extent that the NSPCC is setting up three special centres for them in London alone, this in fact being all it can afford. (Legacies to the NSPCC in 1966 totalled £308,600, while those to the RSPCA in the same period were £703,330.)

The plain facts are that an enormous number of dull and resentful people are revoltingly cruel to their children, and a few intelligent people as well. No experimental animal in England suffers to the same extent, and the courts are astonishingly lenient with offenders.

The material presented in this part is not intended to show that *all* human beings are capable of such behaviour—only that enough of them are to constitute a menace to the eventual elimination of unnecessary pain in any form, from school bullying to nuclear war. We have reached a stage in our existence when the process of evolution itself can to a significant extent be controlled by Man, and it is obviously vital that any such control should be exercised in the right direction. The problems, including that of world over-population, are immense, and their solution must depend very much the attitude of individuals towards them. One attitude that militates against success is thinking that severe pain is an inevitable part of life, with the grim corollary of permitted infliction. In this particular field we have made some progress, for a revolution has taken place since the middle of the last century in methods for the relief of pain and its aura of distress.

PART FOUR

PREVENTION AND RELIEF

IN THIS PART we shall be mainly concerned with the methods devised and used in medical circles, but of course the concept that unnecessary pain should be prevented or eased has a much wider validity than this.

There are theoretically four ways of relieving or preventing pain: removal of the stimulus; interrupting the pain pathways; reducing or abolishing the perception of pain; and altering the emotional attitude towards it. There may be much overlap between these in practice, but the categories are convenient for our particular purpose. It will be appreciated that the subject is a vast one, so that only a few examples can be given of methods in any particular category, enough perhaps to exemplify the principles involved. Methods of treatment before the advent of anaesthesia were not usually aimed primarily at the relief of pain—indeed they were often extremely painful in themselves. We shall therefore mainly consider modern examples, referring to historical work where it is relevant.

The modern doctor faced with a patient in severe pain has three problems: he must relieve suffering; discover the fundamental cause; and do something about this cause. Sometimes the cause is obvious and accessible, such as a splinter under a nail or a decaying tooth; removing it will effect a cure and therefore relieve the pain, though not necessarily immediately. Also the process of removing the cause may itself be painful, calling for sedation or perhaps an anaesthetic.

At other times the cause of the pain is obscure, calling for days or even weeks of careful investigation with complex diagnostic procedures. The eventual treatment may necessitate prolonged drug administration in hospital, or perhaps surgical operations. Relief of pain cannot wait for the successful conclusion of such measures, and indeed they may not be possible; in the great majority of cases special means must be adopted for the purpose of pain relief, initially and in different stages in treatment, if necessary for the rest of the patient's life.

It will be seen that the means of alleviating or preventing pain are usually different from those used for specific treatment of the cause. I think we have now reached the point where relief is invariably possible, but improvement in methods is desirable. Comparatively mild pains are fairly easy to treat, and we have surgical procedures and drugs of great power for the control of intolerable pain due to incurable disease. It is in the intermediate grades such as post-operative pain and pleurisy that our means are far from ideal.

THE AVAILABLE MEANS OF PAIN RELIEF

These include rest, physiotherapy, manipulative methods, counter-irritation, chemical agents, surgery and psychotherapy. It must be admitted at once that the exact mode of action of many of these is not fully understood and, further, that there are frequently psychological overtones of great subtlety whose contribution is hard to assess.

It is in fact very rarely that pain is treated with a single agent; even the apparently simple action of swallowing a couple of aspirins for an ordinary headache is usually combined with rest and with temporary easing of psychic pressures.

Rest

This subject was examined in some detail when dealing with the functions of pain and we saw how often natural healing takes place under the rest enforced by pain. This brings to light one of the many difficulties that attend medical or surgical treatment; for if you abolish pain, by drugs or other means, the protection afforded by nature is lost and further damage may occur. Thus if the pain of coronary disease is suppressed with drugs of the morphine type the patient may feel able to take normal exercise and so completely over-strain an already damaged heart; therefore rest has to be strictly enforced and closely supervised. Rather similar considerations apply to fractures of the long bones. It is easy enough to abolish all pain in a simple fracture of the femur (thigh bone) by injecting a local anaesthetic solution such as procaine between the broken ends. In the absence of immediate proper splinting the patient can then attempt movements that might easily result in serious local damage, even enough to force a bone end through the skin. Nevertheless rest, both to the injured or diseased part and to the patient himself is perhaps the most important single factor in the relief of pain, and we go to considerable lengths to achieve it. Of particular importance in this connection is the question of sleep; a distressing feature of pain is its inevitable exaggeration in the silence and darkness of night, with a vicious circle effect that inhibits natural sleep. This is seriously exhausting, a fact recognized from very early times. One of the most potent methods of persuading obstinate people to part with information or to change their views was (and is) simply to keep them from sleeping by any convenient method; sixty hours is apparently the usual limit. The great French military surgeon Ambroise Paré (1510–1590), who practised in the field of battle for over forty years, said: 'There is nothing that abateth so much the strength as paine.'

Physiotherapy

Literally physiotherapy means the treatment of disease by natural means, a rather loose definition hardly substantiated by the equip-ment in the Physiotherapy Department at a modern hospital. Under the present heading is included every kind of massage and nearly all local applications of gentle heat and cold whether applied pro-fessionally or not.

The use of some of these remedies is practically instinctive. A small child runs to its mother crying, 'I bumped my arm and it hurts!' Rest, physiotherapy and psychotherapy follow instantly: the child is seated on its mother's lap, the arm is gently cradled and soothingly rubbed, and the magic formula 'All better now' chanted repeatedly. No doctor or physiotherapist could better this in efficacy for such minor injuries.

Much of the success of massage and local heat in various forms is due to overcoming muscular spasm – a potent cause of pain. These agents are probably also instrumental in breaking the vicious circle described by Leriche: pain leads to spasm of the muscular walls of small arteries in the part, and this spasm causes further pain. Since arterial pain is caused by stimulation of sympathetic nerve-endings in the vessels themselves the action of such physiotherapy seems to be that of removing the stimulus; much the same action is seen in the use of *radiant heat* and *micro-wave diathermy* for the stiffness following injuries. The diathermy is singularly effective because it heats the tissues by inducing a current in them, leading to a penetrating warmth, very different from the almost completely superficial heat provided by infra-red and radiant-heat appliances.

In itself such heat is only effective for a short time, perhaps an hour after application. Its value lies in enabling the patient to put a joint through an increased range of movement, so stretching the muscles and overcoming spasm. Most of the ointments prescribed for 'rheumatics' and other local pains contain a mild counter-irritant, but much of their effect is due to the massage employed during application.

Quite a lot of muscle spasm with attendant pain is amplified by fear and anxiety, leading to another kind of vicious circle. The skilled physiotherapist encourages people to relax and then to perform movements not otherwise possible – a form of treatment of the utmost value for patients terrified of making the slightest effort after operations, and therefore liable to get chest complications from sheer lack of proper breathing. It is very remarkable how much apparent pain can be overcome by such means, especially in cases where over-sedation would be highly dangerous. Here we have a clear example of the fourth category in the list – the pain itself is presumably unchanged in its essential character, but the patient's attitude towards it is altered so that it becomes acceptable.

Cold

Lowering the temperature of the whole or parts of the body has applications varying from putting a scorched finger under the cold tap to the use of profound hypothermia in heart operations. The use of cold in anaesthesia will be mentioned later.

The *sudden* application of cold objects (whether liquid or solid) to the body surface can be extremely unpleasant and even acutely painful. Slow cold has a numbing effect, even when carried to the extreme of frostbite, but the recovery from this condition is attended by great pain. Cold slowly or gently applied seems to have a specific effect on pain nerve-endings, eventually raising the threshold to vanishing point so that the skin is completely without sensation of any kind.

In view of the obvious and immediate easing of the pain from burns given by a simple application of cold water it does seem quite extraordinary that this has not been the immediate treatment at all times. Yet practically everything else has been preferred by the experts; in forty years of medicine the nearest emergency treatment to cold water I have seen recommended was cold tea, and that was not because of the cold but because of the tannin, which in fact is fortunately present in completely ineffective amounts. The number of special ointments and dressings advised and used, including tannic acid and other coagulation methods that in the past ruined so many hands, must run into hundreds. Some of these nowadays are very effective in easing pain, quelling infections and promoting healing, but it is very interesting indeed to see a quite recent revival of the cold water régime, with the statistic-backed claim that it is not only highly effective in easing pain but also increases the rate of healing and reduces the morbidity of severe burns. It would therefore appear that the instinctive rush for the cold tap and dressings continuously soaked in cold water is completely vindicated by modern research as an emergency treatment for almost any kind of burn, and I strongly recommend it.

People suffering from certain types of constrictive arterial disease often get severe pain in their hands and feet, especially at night, and they usually discover for themselves that the pain is lessened by keeping the affected limb outside the bedclothes. One further example of therapeutic cold is the use of evaporating lotions in bruises and sprains; the part is cooled and so eased. At one time the 'ice bag' was in common use for headaches and other ailments, but seems to lack scientific appeal for moderns.

Manipulative Methods

This is rather controversial ground, because of its association with various unqualified practitioners. A few specialists in Physical Medicine have made a deep study of manipulation on rational grounds, and in their hands the method is both successful and safe so long as a correct diagnosis has been made. Certain medically qualified osteopaths have attained such manipulative skill that their services are in demand by orthodox doctors for their own back-aches, but manipulation of spines by people without medical knowledge can have sinister results—eleven cases of complete paralysis below the waist were so caused in France alone in 1965. Informed and skilled manipulation can sometimes produce instant cure of joint pains that have resisted all other efforts for months.

Counter-Irritants

The principle of substituting one kind of pain for another is very ancient indeed. It was certainly recognized by Hippocrates (fifth century BC) who recommended biting the lip when pain was inevitable. In the Middle Ages one precept was 'diseases not curable by iron are curable by fire'. As we have already seen, duplicating a painful stimulus does not double the total pain; experimental work shows that under normal conditions the presence of pain in one part of the body raises the threshold for pain elsewhere. Whether this is purely a matter of attention or not is uncertain, but the facts are undoubted and most people have experienced episodes of the kind. However, counter-irritants may have a completely different physical effect on occasions; under The Autonomic Nervous System we saw how pain from an internal organ, conveyed by sympathetic nerves, could be felt in an area of skin sending pain nerves to the same segment of the spinal cord. The artificial production of some other sensation in this skin area, such as the burning caused by a mustard-plaster, can not only cancel the visceral pain (if it is not too severe) but may even modify the reaction of the organ itself, possibly by relieving spasm. A good many old-fashioned remedies probably had this dual effect, plus the inevitable psychological factor, and one sometimes feels that a little comfort has been lost in the modern flood of injections and other products of applied science.

A very interesting example of the principles outlined here is the ancient Chinese system known as 'acupuncture' which dates from at least 3,000 BC. Like a good many other unorthodox methods of treatment it can claim some spectacular results, and as usual there is a tendency in certain quarters to make extravagant statements at the expense of ordinary current medical practice. No one can deny that cure of difficult cases is sometimes achieved by such means. Quite apart from the purely psychological aspects inevitably attendant upon fringe medicine we see in acupuncture exemplification of the dual physical process outlined above; the raised threshold of the second pain, and possible modification of a sympathetically innervated root cause.

Fringe Medicine

In this connection a great many people find it difficult to understand why orthodox medicine cannot accept the various fringe branches like acupuncture, chiropractic, Christian Science, 'Black Boxes', spirit healing and herbalism in spite of undoubted (and much publicized) cures when all else has failed. The brief answer is that most of these pursuits have no scientific or even rational foundation; indeed their entire theory can often be summarized in a single sentence. You can set up as a faith healer tomorrow if you wish; there is nothing to stop you. It may be remarked however that the kind of personality required for success in this field is extremely uncommon; these people have the ability to cause interruption of the pain pathway at the highest level by means that are only dimly understood by anyone. If you have this ability, with complete faith in your power to exercise it, and put yourself over with an assurance rarely possible for those having orthodox training, you will obtain the same results in certain difficult cases as other similar practitioners.

If, however, you want to get on the Medical Register you will have to start collecting 'O' levels at the age of fifteen or sixteen; proceed to at least three 'A' levels (or their equivalent), including biology or zoology, physics and chemistry; be one of the fortunate ten per cent selected for entry to a medical school; undergo a course of instruction in anatomy, physiology, pharmacology and bio-chemistry that changes from year to year with advancing knowledge based on continual research; pass difficult examinations in all these subjects after two years of study; begin your theoretical and practical training in pathology, bacteriology, medicine, surgery (including many special branches), gynaecology, obstetrics, psychiatry, public health and forensic medicine; pass very searching written and *viva-voce* examinations in all these subjects at the end of a further three years; obtain posts in a recognized hospital as pre-registration house officers (the most junior doctor), two separate appointments of six months each. You may then (and only then) apply for registra-tion, and once registered you may become an ordinary general practitioner, initially as a trainee. If you want to become a con-sultant in one of the specialties, such as surgery, it will take another five years of unremitting study and training with further (and very hard) examinations to pass. At the end of this time you will begin to know something about your chosen career; and during a life-time of practice it is vitally necessary to keep in close touch with current developments, ready at any time to reject cherished views and favourite methods for more advanced techniques. (The course of study and training leading to medical qualifications and specializa-tion is essentially similar in most countries today.)

Even the very superficial survey of the mechanism of pain in the earlier part of this book shows its manifold possible causes — some extremely obscure. One of the rock-like foundations of medicine today is precise diagnosis, and as we have seen this may take weeks of skilled investigation. If the cause of the pain in your foot is a small tumour pressing on a nerve within the vertebral column, it may be possible for a specially trained surgeon to find this and remove it before irretrievable damage is done.

Most unqualified practitioners have no scientific training and no knowledge of disease processes; with the exception of a few manipulative workers they have no manual skills. They exercise careful selection of cases, specializing in hysterical or neurotic disorders, or in chronic painful conditions that have 'been given up by the doctors'. I am not in any way belittling these sad cases – indeed they are by far the most intractable kind we see: and the fact remains that occasionally the most arrant quack will achieve a spectacular cure where the entire resources of a major teaching hospital have failed to relieve a man's pain. Such cures are almost invariably based on some powerful psychological readjustment, but this merely shows that in such fields we still have a great deal to learn – and unfortunately we cannot learn anything from the author of the cure because he knows even less about the mechanism than we do.

Some further observations on the psychological control of pain will be found at the end of this part.

CHEMICAL AGENTS

These include a very large number of substances used for the control of pain, including local applications, injections, the various drugs given by mouth, and the entire armamentarium of modern anaesthesia. Nearly all this is very recent. A hundred and fifty years ago there were virtually two drugs, and two only, that could be used specifically for the control of pain – opium and alcohol; both had been available for thousands of years – indeed alcohol, formed naturally by the fermentation of vegetable matter with airborne yeasts, was probably discovered by man in the Stone Age.[1] Yet there is a curious scarcity of reference to either product in the old medical literature. One might imagine that every candidate for pre-anaesthetic surgery would have been given a few drinks beforehand, alcohol

[1] *A Man May Drink*, Richard Serjeant.

being plentiful and cheap, but the literature suggests that this was exceptional even in men.

By way of contrast, an approximate count of current British ethical proprietary preparations (i.e. branded products not advertised to the public) shows ninety-four analgesics, ninety-three sedatives and tranquillizers, forty-seven hypnotics, fifty-nine gastro-intestinal sedatives, eighteen muscle relaxants (including those used in anaesthesia), and twenty-nine local and general anaesthetic agents other than chloroform, ether and nitrous oxide gas. Of course many of these preparations have a similar basis, but the choice is wide. Their multiplicity exemplifies imperfection.

In view of the diversity of this subject the drugs used in anaesthesia will be considered first, followed by examples of the numerous other drugs and agents used for the control of pain.

General Anaesthesia

Though alcohol and opium were occasionally used in the past to reduce the pain of operations, neither is in fact powerful enough to do so substantially without great risk. Apart from drugs, attempts have been made at intervals to induce general anaesthesia by hitting the patient on the jaw, or to produce local anaesthesia by compression of limbs with tourniquets, neither very successfully. The first reference to the possibility of surgical anaesthesia by inhalation was in 1800 by the twenty-year-old Humphrey Davy experimenting with *nitrous oxide* (a gas discovered by Priestley in 1772). He inhaled it himself, found it greatly eased his toothache, and suggested it might be of use in surgery. We have no record that the gas was so used for the next forty years, though it was inhaled at parties for 'kicks' often enough. *Ether* was also being inhaled for similar reasons in 1840, and a dental extraction was performed under ether in 1842 by a Dr Clark of Rochester, USA. From then on various people made experiments with nitrous oxide and ether, and the first authentic demonstration of surgical anaesthesia was probably when a neck tumour was removed at the Massachusetts General Hospital by John Collins Warren, under ether anaesthesia administered by a dentist, William Morton, on October 16th 1846.

Thus a means was at last found by which the fearful pain of surgical operations could be completely abolished with comparative ease and certainty. The discovery of chloroform quickly followed that of ether, and for the next eighty or ninety years these two agents, with nitrous oxide, were the only substances used for many thousands of operations. Chloroform was more pleasant to inhale than ether, and had other advantages in the achievement of painless labour. The preposterous religious objections to its use in obstetrics ceased abruptly when Queen Victoria was given it in 1853, and it became known as *anaesthesia à la Reine*.

There have been several advances in gases and volatile liquids for anaesthesia, the additions being the gas *cyclopropane; vinyl ether, ethyl chloride* (both only suited to very short cases); *trichlorethylene*, which can be used for long periods but produces no relaxation (and incidentally is ideal for removing grease stains from clothes); and *halothane* (1.1, 1–triflouro–2, 2–bromochlorethane) which is non-inflammable and fairly pleasant to inhale. Modern techniques make little use of any but cyclopropane, trichlorethylene and halothane, and the once-familiar smell of ether in the operating theatre is almost a thing of the past. The main reason for this change has been the introduction of *muscle relaxants* to secure the operating conditions required by the surgeon. Achieving this state with ether meant a dangerously deep state of unconsciousness; the patients took a very long time to come round afterwards; chest complications were rather common; and there was a great tendency towards nausea and vomiting. In addition, many patients disliked or were frightened by the application of a mask over the face for induction, particularly when associated with the rather pungent smell of ether. These were small prices to pay for painless surgery, but improvements were greatly needed.

The first major improvement was the introduction of anaesthetics that could be given by injection into a vein in the 1930's. These are mainly used to induce the initial sleep, anaesthesia being continued through a mask or tube. Thiopentone is the main example.

In 1938 the second major advance came in the form of a *muscle-relaxant* based on the ancient South American arrow poison *curare*, which paralysed victims without killing them. We now have a wide choice of these relaxants; they are very safe in skilled hands, but they

5

paralyse *all* voluntary muscles, including those of respiration, so the patient has to be connected to a bag that can be squeezed or to a machine that does his breathing for him. Sleep need only be quite light, and the anaesthetist has very complete control.

Recent major developments have been those in anaesthetics and surgery which have made long operations on the heart possible. The patient's blood can be completely diverted from his heart and lungs and pumped through machines that supply it with oxygen, remove carbon dioxide, and *cool* it to a point at which all cellular activity in the body apparently ceases, including that of the brain itself. These patients are dead by any known test – their pulse and breathing has stopped, they are cold, and an electroencephalogram (brain-waves) shows no response. Yet after hours of intricate work, perhaps replacing a damaged heart-valve, or even the heart itself, the blood is re-warmed, circulates once more through the lungs, heart and brain and the patient comes to life aparently unchanged. How long it will ultimately be possible to continue this 'profound hypothermia' is not certain, but it is definitely included among the various schemes that may make voyages lasting many years to the stars possible. The other fascinating possibility already under serious consideration is that of going into deep-freeze hibernation and being wakened a number of years later, perhaps when the cure for your 'incurable' disease has been found. The old dream of waking up every hundred years to have a look round also begins to look feasible.

Latest developments are confining the profound hypothermia to the heart itself, the rest of the body, including the brain, being at normal temperature.

Fully controlled inhalation anaesthesia combined with muscle relaxants has reduced the hazards of surgery to the point where we rarely refuse operation to anyone on the grounds of age, and not often on general condition if this cannot be improved in the time available.

Local, Regional and Spinal Anaesthesia

There has been little real progress in this field since 1940 or so, mainly because the development of general anaesthetics has made it

largely unnecessary for major work. *Surface applications* in the form
of solutions or ointments of cocaine-like substances are useful in
numbing mucous membranes in the mouth or throat, or to relieve
the pain in raw skin surfaces from ulcers or burns. They act directly
on nerve endings.

The whole system of local anaesthesia probably began in 1884,
when Carl Koller in Vienna used a solution of cocaine for a small
eye operation. Some years later the production of fine hollow needles
enabled surgeons to inject cocaine derivatives under the skin, producing complete numbness in that area, a method probably first
used by William Stewart Halsted in about 1890 at the Johns
Hopkins Hospital in Baltimore.

Regional anaesthesia is achieved by allowing these agents to act
upon the sensory nerves themselves, with the result of numbing
the entire area supplied. Thus we can anaesthetize a finger or a toe
by injecting a solution of procaine hydrochloride around its base,
blocking the two digital nerves; the resulting anaesthesia lasts
about half an hour, and enables us to remove nails or repair injuries
without the slightest discomfort in a fully conscious patient. By
careful selection of injection sites almost any area of the body can
be anaesthetized in this way. With scrupulous technique special
solutions can be injected round the spinal cord itself by passing a
needle between the vertebrae, producing not only anaesthesia at the
chosen level (abdominal, pelvic, lower limb) but complete muscular
relaxation as well. This *spinal anaesthesia*, though providing perfect
operating conditions, carries risks of its own, and since the introduction of muscle-relaxants has become very much less popular. Local
and regional anaesthesia is still extensively used for dentistry, eye
operations, and minor surgery in hospital out-patients departments.
A technique known as 'caudal block' affecting the perineum only, is
much used in obstetrics.

The various anaesthetic agents discussed so far act either by
interrupting pain pathways (local, regional or spinal) or by cancelling
the perception of pain (general anaesthesia). A very subtle method
has been developed which appears to act partially at the highest
level – by modifying the patient's attitude towards pain. Known
as *neuroleptanalgesia* it produces a curious semi-cataleptic state –

almost like an artificial hibernation – and this is combined with analgesic drugs of quite moderate power. Though rather dreamy these patients are conscious and able to talk, yet appear indifferent to surgical procedures of some magnitude. By this means it is possible to operate on people who would be impossibly bad risks by almost any other method; we have seen a man of ninety, with chronic heart failure, advanced bronchitis and diabetes, whose leg was successfully amputated for a gangrenous foot under neuro-leptanalgesia.

One alternative in extremely bad-risk cases is the employment of the numbing effects of *cold*; it is in fact possible to amputate a man's leg painlessly after it has been packed round with ice for some hours. The indications for this procedure are however becoming very rare.

Analgesics

These drugs, usually known as 'pain killers', have been the subject of a great deal of research, but the ideal has yet to be found; no drug exists that will control severe pain without penalty.

Aspirin, either alone or in combination with other drugs, is by far the commonest analgesic substance in use today. It was first used medically by Herman Dresser in 1893, and although comparatively mild for general use has a specific action of rather more power in the joint pains associated with rheumatism. There are few toxic effects in ordinary doses, though a tendency to gastric ulceration has been noted, especially if the tablets are swallowed whole. The combination of aspirin with steroids, effective symptomatically in some cases of advanced rheumatoid arthritis, can cause enormous gastric ulcers that may even perforate with very little pain, leading to some tricky problems in diagnosis and management. Hardly a house in the civilized world is without some kind of aspirin, usually in the unnecessarily expensive much-advertised brands. Its consumption for minor aches and pains is prodigious, the annual world output at present being in the region of 30,000 tons.

Morphine, at almost the other end of the scale in power, is certainly the most widely used of the strong analgesic drugs. First isolated from raw opium in 1806 it had to wait for the hollow needle to exhibit its real might—and of this there is no doubt. There are very few pains so intense that they are not rendered tolerable by the first injection of morphine, and an exhausted sufferer can sink into sleep at last. It has the further valuable effect of allaying anxiety. These properties render it almost indispensable in medical practice, but there are considerable drawbacks to its use.

Some people would definitely prefer pain to the side-effects that morphine has on them—an intense depression associated with waves of nausea and sometimes vomiting. Even when these symptoms are minimal morphine has to be given in sharply increasing doses to remain effective, and patients rapidly become completely dependent upon it. Moreover a further set of distressing symptoms follows its withdrawal. In other words, it is a drug of addiction, and therefore must usually be reserved for the 'once only' indication—such as immediately after painful operations—or where incurable and rapidly advancing disease is causing great pain, and neither the size of dose nor addiction are of any consequence. Morphine is also used to secure essential rest in certain cases of heart disease. There is a tendency nowadays to avoid morphine whenever possible, but in some circumstances it is irreplaceable because of its sheer power over pain.

Heroin (diacetylmorphine) was first developed in an attempt to overcome the disadvantages of morphine; it was found to be about five times as powerful and hence completely unequalled as a pain-killer. It also unfortunately proved to be unequalled as a drug of addiction, to such a degree that its manufacture is wholly forbidden in the USA. In spite of such restrictions at least half of all American drug-addicts are taking heroin, and traffic in the drug constitutes a major world problem. Its withdrawal from our own pharmacopoeia is opposed by many of the profession who have any contact with the terminal stages of some growths and similar cases; they feel that the relief of agony should not be prejudiced by psychopaths and by the ineptitude of Governments.

However a good deal of research is being devoted to finding very powerful drugs for the relief of pain without undesirable side-effects, and some of these do show promise. The most powerful so far is known as 'Bentley's compound' after its British discoverer, and is approximately ten thousand times as strong as morphine. Marshall

Gates[1] reports that it has been used to subdue wild elephants in an African game-reserve, the dose being one milligram per elephant. Unfortunately it is an intense respiratory depressant and therefore contra-indicated in Medicine. A quite different series of compounds is derived from the *benzorphans*; *cyclorphan* and *cyclazocine* seem to be non-addicting and non-depressant, but produce hallucinations in therapeutic doses, while *pentazocine* is non-addicting and non-hallucinatory, but is not completely free from side effects. So we do seem to be on the brink of discovering a non-addicting, non-hallucinatory and non-depressant drug with the analgesic power of heroin. After it has been produced, and thoroughly tested, we can gladly abandon morphine and heroin altogether.

A large and increasing number of preparations with potency between morphine and aspirin suit some people and not others, so that finding the right pill is often a matter of trial and error.

The mode of action of analgesics is not by any means fully known and probably varies considerably with different drugs. Morphine seems to act partly by blocking the pathways at a high level and partly by altering the emotional response. One rather curious feature is that morphine and allied narcotic drugs will control severe established pain, but have little or no effect on the threshold for sharp superficial injuries such as stabs with a needle. Other drugs appear to reduce perception in a manner rather like small doses of nitrous oxide or large doses of alcohol.

In view of the complexity of the pain reaction it is hardly surprising that the assessment of analgesic drugs is difficult. The American anaesthetist, Henry K. Beecher,[2] found in very extended trials that in post-operative and other kinds of pain due to injury or disease an injection of sterile saline (which is completely without any pharmacological action) was as effective as the usual dose of morphine in 35 per cent of cases. This figure is surprisingly high, but certainly illustrates just once again the very large psychological factors that contribute to our experience of pain; in *experimental* pain this use of inert substances (known as 'placebos') is only effective in 3.2 per cent of cases. This kind of test is carefully controlled on the 'double-blind' system—neither the patient nor the

---

[1] 'Analgesic Drugs', in *Scientific American*, November, 1966.
[2] *Pain, an International Symposium*, ed. R. S. Knighton and P. Dumke.

person actually giving the injection knows what is in the syringe. One should also perhaps mention that if the *placebo* fails the patient is given the real thing without delay.

Tranquillizers

The enormous use of these drugs outside the field of mental disease (for which they were originally developed) is a reflection of the unrest of our time. Although they have no specific effect on the perception of physical pain their action of allaying anxiety and reducing emotional response leads to their widespread prescription for certain types of people in pain. It must be obvious that emotionally unstable people are just as likely as anyone else to get serious organic diseases, including those that cause pain. Surgical operations tend to focus attention upon some part of the body, if only because of the presence of a visible scar. The emotionally labile remain very much aware of this, sometimes for many years, and occasionally succeed in confusing doctors to the extent of performing further operations for 'adhesions' and so on when none exist. It is by no means easy to be certain of the diagnosis in such cases, the main reason being that few pains are exclusively psychogenic, so that some physical basis, however small, usually exists as well. Some of these secondary operations do disclose a causative adhesion, and the patient recovers – and so do quite a number of patients in whom no abnormality was found. There is no doubt that the chronic worriers are helped by small doses of tranquillizing drugs, also that they become dependent upon them. Of course such people do not confine their clinical recitals to medical audiences, and the exhibition of tranquillizers may well make life more tolerable and less boring not only for their doctors, but also for their relations and friends.

There is little doubt that these tranquillizing drugs have been avidly seized upon in some quarters as a heaven-sent short cut for the suppression of symptoms with a 'nuisance value', and may have much the same effect as a time-consuming and uncertain psychoanalysis – that of converting troublesome cases into what one American internist calls 'castrated cretins'.[1]

[1] 'Psychosomatic Medicine', the First Hahnemann Symposium (quoting Leo E. Hollister, M.D.).

The wise and informed use of these new drugs has enabled thousands of people to live almost normal lives who would not so long ago have been confined under wretched conditions in one of our enormous mental hospitals. In addition, their action is being closely studied and this is adding to our total knowledge of the mind.

It is sometimes forgotten that alcohol and tobacco have a remarkably tranquillizing effect, and the results of enforced withdrawal are not easy to estimate — a number of us would become completely insufferable.

Muscle Relaxants

In addition to the powerful muscle relaxants referred to under Anaesthesia there is a further group of drugs having the specific effect of relaxing the spasm of plain muscle — the muscle in the walls of organs and arteries. These are useful for controlling pain from such sources, but the origin of this kind of pain is often rather complex and consequently one cannot necessarily control it by any single method. Examples are the pain of *intermittent claudication* with cramp in the calf — sometimes this is due to spasm of arteries supplying the muscles, and can be relieved by drugs; *angina pectoris*, when caused by spasm of the coronary arteries, specifically terminated by the inhalation of amyl nitrite; *intestinal colic*, for which some complex organic compounds have been devised; and the severe colics caused by stones in the biliary and urinary systems, often requiring morphine for relief, but aided by pethidine, atropine and other drugs with a strong effect in relaxing plain muscle.

A great many drugs are also marketed having a relaxing effect on ordinary skeletal (voluntary) muscle, and sometimes these help in muscle strain and other painful conditions in which spasm is a feature.

Antibiotics and Sulphonamides

These drugs, which have revolutionized Medicine since the 1930's, have a specific inhibiting effect on bacteria and enable us to control many diseases that were formerly fatal. Their primary purpose is not to relieve pain, but a number of the conditions we treat with them are intrinsically painful, and the ease that follows within an hour or so of the first dose is often dramatic, constituting an excellent example of controlling pain by treatment of the cause.

Endocrines

Originally derived from male and female sex-glands and from the adrenal glands, these now have many synthetic counterparts of great potency. Reference has already been made to the use of steroids for rheumatoid arthritis. Other painful conditions that can be treated or relieved with steroids, cortico-steroids and allied compounds include dysmenorrhoea, (painful menstruation), advanced breast cancer, prostatic cancer, and various painful joint and tendon disorders. An example of rather subtle pain therapy is the injection treatment of 'tennis elbow', a condition that has always proved obstinately difficult to cure. It was found that the injection of a particular cortico-steroid sometimes eased the pain after a few days, but at the expense of an extremely painful injection and very great discomfort for some time afterwards. Combining the cortico-steroid with a local anaesthetic (procaine) made the injection and the period immediately afterwards tolerable, but success was limited by the difficulty of getting the injected fluid to reach the whole affected area. Finally a substance called *hyaluronidase* was devised which has the action of diffusing injected fluid through tissues, and this added to the cortico-steroid and procaine resulted in a combination that often permanently cures the pain of tennis-elbow and allied conditions with a single injection.

Finally in this category reference must be made to the treatment of certain malignant diseases with radiation, and with the complex and tricky *cytotoxic drugs*. Once again these are not used specifically for the relief of pain but often have this result by modifying the local effects of the growth.

This review of drugs and other chemical agents is only intended to give some idea of the vastness of the field, and incidentally of the necessity to arrive at a correct diagnosis of the cause of the pain and to select a drug from the appropriate group for its treatment. There is considerable scope for improvement in drugs specifically for pain relief. What is sought is an agent that acts directly on the thalamic relay-centres in the mid-brain; whose potency depends purely on the dose; which has no side-effects in any dosage; that does not require ever-increasing amounts; that is available in short- and long-acting forms; and, preferably, that is cheap. Should such a drug ever be discovered it will have profound effects, not only on Medicine but perhaps on the whole future of the human race and the course of evolution. Not all these effects will be beneficial, particularly if it gets out of medical control and becomes exploited commercially. It might even be disastrous.

THE SURGICAL RELIEF OF PAIN

The operations of surgery can lead to relief of pain in a number of ways, some resulting in elimination of the original disease, some designed purely to interrupt nerve pathways where every other means has failed. The large majority of people seen by surgeons are originally referred by their general practitioners because of conditions causing pain; and in most of these we are fortunately able to deal with a fairly obvious cause in a reasonably straightforward manner. The pain may be due to an abscess, a hernia, piles, varicose veins, a grumbling appendix, a carious tooth, a deformed toe, a cystic ovary, a blocked sinus, a gallstone. It is usually (not always) a comparatively simple matter to deal with these complaints and restore our patients to normal, though possibly lacking a tooth or some other small part. Other abnormalities may require major surgery for their correction — removal of the uterus (womb), or the stomach, or a leg, or reconstruction of a hip joint, or ligature of an aneurysm within the skull; here we may leave a patient handicapped in various ways, but free from pain and from the original disease.

In a third group a condition is found, perhaps a growth, which cannot be removed or has spread to distant parts of the body. For these we may find surgical ways of relieving our patient's pain by careful selective removal of a tumour, or by-passing the affected organ. Some of these operations lead to complete symptomatic relief for quite long periods even if the original condition was malignant in nature, and they may be life-saving in the sense of averting immediate death, as in the case of acute intestinal obstruction due to an irremovable cancer of the bowel, treated by a simple short-circuit procedure.

In all these operations we are very much concerned with the actual cause of the pain – we attempt to remove it, or if that is not possible to by-pass it.

There is however a fourth group of cases in which the entire object of surgery is to relieve pain and no attempt is made to deal with the primary cause. Most of these operations entail interference with the neurological pathways of pain described in Part I, and some of them offer the only way of controlling intolerable pain in hopeless diseases without drugging the patient into stupidity.

Nerve Endings

It is possible to isolate nerve endings from the terminal fibrils of sensory nerves by raising a thin flap of skin and then sewing it back again like a graft. This method is only of service when pain originates in the skin itself and there are nearly always better methods of attack.

Cutting Nerves

It might be imagined that a simple way of easing severe pain in a limb or a joint would be to divide the main sensory nerves to the part. The method was probably first practised by Victor Horsley in 1873. It has several serious disadvantages: it deprives the skin of all sensation, so that an area of complete numbness results, and this is not only unpleasant for the patient but also makes the numb area more susceptible to injury; in addition if the pain is in any way connected with local blood vessels it will not necessarily be relieved, since pain from these is conveyed in sympathetic nerves initially in the walls of the vessels themselves. Occasionally a severe pain arises as a result of disease in a fairly small peripheral nerve which can be cut or removed; the resulting loss of sensation is small because of overlap by neighbouring nerves. Success is achieved by this method for intense pain in the outer side of the thigh, and in special areas of the front and back of the scalp. Severe neuralgia in large nerves such as the Trigeminal, causing *tic-doloreux*, is treated by injection or surgical section of special parts of the nerve containing the sensory fibres. The greatest care is taken to preserve sensation in the surface of the eye, otherwise the blink reflex is lost. Occasionally this is unavoidable, and the eye has to be protected from harm by almost closing the lids with fine stitches until the reflex returns—a process that may take six months.

Visceral Nerve Section

The modern treatment of duodenal ulcer includes interrupting the *vagus nerves*, combined with a simple by-pass or short-circuit procedure. This is not done just because these nerves convey pain sensations but because they control the mobility and the acid secretion in the stomach, and both factors play a part in ulcer pain.

Partially Injured Nerves

Arm and leg injuries sometimes result in a form of neuritis in the median or sciatic nerves giving rise to the intense burning pain (with redness and sweating) known as *causalgia*. If the nerve is being pressed on, it can be freed, but in late stages much of the pain arises from peripheral arteries and is accordingly not relieved by attack on the nerve itself. Moreover direct interference in the form of injection or partial section is likely to affect the fibres controlling muscles (motor fibres), with resulting paralysis. Alleviation can however sometimes be achieved by *sympathectomy*, and certain other surgical measures.

Sympathectomy

Interruption of the autonomic nervous system was probably first suggested in 1899. It was practised by Leriche in 1916 for causalgia, but his method was to strip the outer coat off the main artery of the limb on the assumption that this would interrupt the sympathetic innervation below that level and so relax the vessels and cut the pain pathway. Leriche himself appears to have had a number of successes but other people could not achieve the same results with his methods. Later, when more exact anatomy disclosed definite sympathetic nerve fibres in the neck and thorax and abdomen, much more positive results were obtained; they are however still rather unpredictable, and on the whole sympathectomy is regarded more as an adjuvant to other measures than as a pain-relieving operation in its own right. It has been successfully used in the cramp-like pains of *intermittent claudication* (pain in the calf and limping due to arterial disease), for threatened gangrene of the toes (particularly in elderly people), for the pain and skin changes following frostbite, and for some forms of angina pectoris.

Operations on the Spinal Cord

We saw in Part I how the nerve fibres conveying the sense of pain travel upwards in the spinal cord to reach the brain. These tracts can be very accurately located, and using extremely careful technique can be divided with a tiny knife after exposing the cord in its vertebral canal from the back (laminectomy). These operations are rather hazardous and may carry possible penalties in the form of partial anaesthesia and paralysis or spasm of local muscles, but they can occasionally offer relief for the intolerable pain of some advanced malignant growths without the use of drugs. One particular operation has proved that the fine sensation of *light touch* in the skin is quite distinct from the sensations of *temperature and pain* which travel up the spinal cord towards the thalamus (and other centres) in a small bundle known as the *spino-thalamic tract*. Division of this tract alone can leave the patient with the sense of light touch — and incidentally with his withdrawal reflex intact — but completely free from the pain.

Once within the vertebral column one or more of the *sensory nerve roots* can be divided, leading to anaesthesia in the part supplied. A modification of this is to inject an oily solution of *phenol* into the vertebral canal, rather like a spinal anaesthetic is given. The phenol seems to have a partially selective action on sensory fibres while sparing motor ones, so the pain is diminished without causing paralysis, but the exact distribution is difficult to control and calls for skilled handling under X-ray guidance.

Pre-frontal Leucotomy

The enormous frontal lobes of the human brain contain millions of nerve cells and association fibres, yet their exact function is unknown. They can be removed or their connections with the rest of the brain severed, without affecting any sensation or any motor power. Yet a man's reactions, his emotions and his social behaviour are subtly altered; he becomes more placid, accepts adverse situations, changes his sense of values. Some of these effects help in cases of profound alteration in personality or where obsession with severe pain exists. After pre-frontal leucotomy a man is said to feel exactly the same pain but not to care about it — it other words it has altered his attitude towards pain in a manner previously only considered possibly by the application of some form of psychotherapy.

Stereotactic Surgery

Some of the most exacting and intricate of all surgical operations are being used for the relief of pain from incurable disease, and are aimed at the thalamus itself and other nuclei and fibres in the deep interior of the brain. These centres are being attacked with proton beams, radio-frequency heat, cryogenic local cold and even ultrasound, aimed with millimetre accuracy by precision apparatus anchored to the skull itself.

It should be mentioned however that the primary purpose of stereotactic surgery is not the relief of pain but the alleviation of mental symptoms such as intense chronic depression, and that some remarkable cures have been obtained in patients confined to mental hospitals for years, all other treatment having failed.

Hormone Surgery

Some kinds of malignant disease are associated in a very subtle manner with the secretions of the ductless glands – the hormones – and in a rather empirical way the most advanced stages of these growths, involving wide and distant spread, can be modified by hormone manipulation. The particular growths involved are those of breast, prostate, ovary and testis. It has been found that sometimes marked regression of secondary deposits, and often immense relief from pain, follows surgical removal of the adrenal glands or of the pituitary gland. These operations (adrenalectomy and hypophysectomy) are difficult and dangerous, particularly in people debilitated by the effects of advanced cancer, but the results are occasionally dramatic, and accordingly the risk may be well worth taking.

PSYCHOTHERAPY

Repeated reference has been made in previous parts to the psychological aspects of pain and to the manner in which it can be grossly exaggerated or totally cancelled by purely mental processes. Normally such phenomena are beyond our control except in very minor degrees, and they depend on the operation of imponderables like fear and faith. The very fact that they work implies the possibility of voluntary control, either by the individual or by someone else, but one encounters many examples that exemplify the uncertainty of the process as ordinarily applied.

A woman of fifty goes to a surgeon complaining of a painful lump in her breast. She has had it for months, but has only just seen the doctor about it. The pain is incessant, it keeps her awake at night, interferes with her work, ruins her appetite. She has lost weight and looks haggard. Examination quickly reveals a simple non-malignant condition requiring minimal interference.

This patient fears that she has cancer. The flat denial is not usually enough – she has to be told that she was absolutely right to seek advice and that some of these minor breast conditions are very uncomfortable, but she is one of the fortunate ones and does NOT have cancer. (I have seen women nearly faint with relief and burst into tears on hearing this.) Two weeks later she says the pain has almost gone, on treatment that cannot possibly have had any real physical effect; the little lump can be removed at some convenient time later on.

Another patient complains of various abdominal pains in considerable and bizarre detail. A full series of X-rays and other investigations confirm the clinical impression that there is no detectable organic disease. Complete explanation and reassurance result in hostile withdrawal; the pains continue, and after a time the patient ends by seeing a psychiatrist and probably receiving tranquillizers.

Both types of case are common enough in any medical practice and illustrate the diversity of psychogenic pain and its background.

Instruction in Relaxation

A good many mental disciplines are aimed at inducing complete bodily and emotional rest for specified periods during the day, or at will. This is not so easy to achieve as some people imagine, and one constantly encounters patients who simply do not understand what is meant by relaxing their muscles. Reasonably intelligent people can be taught how to do this, and it forms part of Yoga and other cults; its benefits in normal circumstances are not proved, but there is no possible doubt about its value in illness, whether painful or otherwise.

In the particular field of obstetrics the ability to relax completely has been shown by Grantly Dick Read and others to reduce very greatly the amount of pain involved. There are of course other factors here, such as careful explanation of the process of natural birth, resulting in a change of attitude towards it; the loss of fear; and the patient's trust and confidence in those who are looking after her.

Psychiatric Treatment

This implies specialized investigation of the causes underlying behaviour and symptoms, and appropriate treatment. Psychiatry now stands rather in the position of General Medicine in the early 1930's; diagnosis was a highly developed art, treatment was largely empirical, there were almost no specifics – no chemotherapy, no antibiotics, no steroids. Practically, the main advances in psychiatric treatment in the last thirty years have been in social work, in the introduction of tranquillizing and anti-depressant drugs, shock therapy, and the occasional surgical operation. An increasing number of conditions previously considered to be purely mental illnesses now prove to have an organic basis, and some of these nowadays have specific remedies.

It is however a fact that lengthy investigation may disclose suppressed worries and complexes based on correctable conditions, and this does result occasionally in the complete termination of apparently intractable pain – perhaps after months or even years of psychoanalysis.

In the fullness of time we may understand the kind of mental processes involved and even acquire the ability to manipulate them. This will bring a revolution in treatment at least as great as anaesthetics, asepsis and antibiotics; moreover it will have effects in every field of human behaviour.

Hypnosis

We now know that the basic phenomena of hypnosis have been

used for thousands of years, appearing as religious trances, magical cures, fairground fascination and in many other guises. It first attained prominence in its own right as Mesmerism, after Anton Mesmer (1734–1815), a Parisian doctor with a lucrative society practice who produced apparently miraculous effects by hand movements known as 'passes', and thought they were due to a magnetic fluid generated by the operator. Although this theory is now considered archaic one must admit that nothing very substantial has replaced it to account for the phenomena, and these are not trivial by any means, particularly in regard to pain.

The first man to demonstrate this beyond all possible doubt was James Esdaile, who graduated as a doctor at Edinburgh in 1830 and was later appointed Medical Officer to the East India Company. He became interested in Mesmerism, and in 1845 began using it to render the natives unconscious while he performed various operations ranging from lancing boils to amputations and the removal of the enormous scrotal tumours caused by elephantiasis. In the following six years until he left India in 1851 Esdaile performed thousands of minor operations and at least three hundred major ones, completely painlessly, under hypnosis.

The reader might conclude that this pioneer work in painless surgery was acclaimed and its originator loaded with honours. Of course not – his work was sneered at and discredited both in India and at home, but do please notice the dates; he started his fantastic series of operations almost exactly a year *after* the first public demonstration of ether anaesthesia in America, and the news of this spread like wildfire all over the civilized world. Even Esdaile himself was much less successful in his attempts to mesmerize the hard-headed Scots than he had been with the credulous and frightened Indians in Calcutta. The stark *fact* that major surgery had been done painlessly without drugs of any kind was overlooked. Esdaile became disappointed and embittered and died in Scotland at the age of fifty in 1859. The term 'hypnotism' was coined by another doctor, James Braid, in 1842. Since then, through many vicissitudes, hypnosis has been guardedly accepted in the medical profession as having certain limited indications. The big trouble is that one cannot hypnotize everybody – and one cannot predict with certainty who will be affected. Moreover the final effect may be trivial or profound, again unpredictable. At best one may reach the stage of surgical anaesthesia, after perhaps ten half-hour sessions with a sensitive patient. Once attained, there is no doubt whatever about the genuineness of the phenomenon – I have done several operations under hypnotic anaesthesia, including the removal of an appendix; anaesthesia was complete and there was no post-operative pain. The patient was fully conscious and co-operative; he got off the operating table without help, walked back to the ward, slept peacefully for twelve hours and had no pain or even discomfort. *But* he was a proved sensitive who had been hypnotized for demonstration purposes many times, and who just happened to get acute appendicitis.

Hypnosis is particularly successful in the field of dental surgery, when time is available for its practice. Of course in dentistry treatment tends to be prolonged, sometimes over many years, and it may be well worth the initial effort to obtain complete co-operation and relaxation from certain very nervous patients, especially children.

During World War II hypnosis was successfully used by several doctors in prison camps under terrible conditions, with no anaesthetics available, for the performance of various operations and dressings that would otherwise have entailed very severe pain.

Hypnosis is a remarkable and perfectly genuine phenomenon and is worthy of much deeper study. Some of its medical applications in the fields of dentistry and obstetrics are unique, but we cannot depend on it in the way we can on general anaesthetic agents. Its mechanism is obscure, and its image has been distorted in the public eye by historical and stage associations with magic.

The real point here is that *complete indifference to pain can be achieved by purely psychic means* – in other words by a rearrangement of mental processes. I believe this is far more important than any other single factor in the problem of pain, and may possibly hold the clue to its eventual solution.

ELECTRICAL ANAESTHESIA

Before leaving the alleviation of pain I think we should consider the possible future use of electrical anaesthesia. A start has been made with the induction of sleep by suitably placed electrodes on the head, connected to batteries, but one cannot entirely exclude the operation of factors based on credulity rather than currents. However a demonstration has already been given of a cow rendered unconscious by electrical means, after which, 'looking startled and pausing only to soil the carpet', it staggered off apparently none the worse.[1] Already we see suggestions that anaesthetists should be kept out of the operating area, controlling their patients through sleeves rather like the way scientists handle radio-active materials; combined with colour television, electrical methods would seem to promise the possibility of their conducting the entire procedure from home.

THE ULTIMATE RELIEF

Pain of any kind ceases with death – an end craved by countless victims of cruelty, and occasionally carried out as an act of mercy. The suffering from the terminal stages of incurable disease is not confined to pain; it may include complete incontinence, uncontrollable vomiting, inability to move because of fractures in the limbs and spine, and dementia from secondary deposits in the brain. A movement exists to legalize 'mercy killing' (euthanasia) in circumstances of this kind, entailing consent of the patient and relatives, with approval of two doctors, signatures on a 'consent form' and finally the *coup de grâce* by a doctor.

I want to make three observations on this controversial subject.

1. In spite of any statements to the contrary conditions continually occur in which pain and suffering are impossible to control without drugging the patient into insensibility or converting him into a helpless vegetable by other means.

2. In the present state of our social and emotional evolution I do not think that anyone should face the responsibility for signing forms of this nature.

3. Nobody should be allowed to suffer in the way I have described above; moreover it is totally unnecessary. The law allows the control of suffering to the point of measures dangerous to life, and

[1] I much regret my carelessness in losing track of the article containing this elegant description.

most doctors with any compassion in their hearts use them where necessary. It is a mistake to imagine that people have to be murdered to secure release. The entire principle was summarized in two lines by Arthur Hugh Clough:

Thou shalt not kill, but need'st not strive
Officiously to keep alive.

Officiously keeping alive is a terrible thing and should be more vigorously condemned in our medical schools. It includes transfusing patients racked and demented with secondary cancer, and it also includes withholding vast doses of powerful drugs from those who truly need them. Such people should have the right to die in dignity and peace if this is possible, and I conceive it part of my duty as a surgeon to ease their way without signatures on a form by them or their relatives; I also expect the law to protect me in this attitude, and I think it does.

PART FIVE

THE PARADOX OF PAIN

WE HAVE NOW arrived at the final stage in our examination of Pain — a stage of rather severe conflict. Pain has been proved essential to the evolutionary process, yet in its severe degrees it is mostly useless. Men seem to have an innate tendency to cruelty, which leaps into prominence at the slightest chance. The highest virtues such as compassion and pity depend on the existence of pain, and yet the greatest feats of endurance may be associated with superstition and deception.

A recurring theme in fiction, substantiated by a host of facts, is that some painful experiences have a profoundly valuable effect on people's lives. It seems particularly applicable to short violent illnesses or accidents attended by a great deal of pain, but from which the individual recovers completely. Sometimes such an experience shakes a man out of a previously rather torpid existence, makes him realize what he has to be thankful for in normal health, and induces appreciation of the sufferings of others; he surprises himself with unknown reserves of fortitude, and he may even notice acts of kindness and compassion by those looking after him. Patients have told me all these things at times, and have often said 'it taught me a lot'.

When thinking about the enigma of pain in Part III we looked at a good many human characteristics that led directly or indirectly to violence and cruelty. Among these were superstition, hate, jealousy, vengeance, intolerance and greed — and to some degree these are so common as to seem intrinsic parts of human nature. Psychiatric studies show that suspicion and hate are very much more basic than love is, suppressed though they may be. It is of course easy to criticize the behaviour of others. We seem to be terrified of the potential cruelty within us and so to condemn furiously its manifestations outside ourselves. This fury is significant.

Bronowski[1] called it 'looking in the dark mirror', and says: 'We have it in ourselves to be murderers and con-men and perverts and the scum of the earth.'

All rather hopeless. Are there any grounds for optimism?

Man's early environment on Earth must have been an intensely hostile one. He was a small animal, not at all physically strong, and possessing almost nothing in the way of natural defences such as fangs or claws. He survived because the enormous development of his fore-brain enabled him to out-think other creatures, however vicious and however large, to kill them for food, make them work for him, and to herd them or ride them. In order to do these things he had to be immensely suspicious, utterly ruthless and diabolically cunning – and one must accept that these characteristics were 'instinctive' in the sense that they were part of his genetic pattern, like a bird's ability to fly or a seal's to swim.

'The life of man is the life of a brave and splendid, cruel and cunning beast of prey. He lives by catching, killing and consuming. Since he exists, he must be master.'[2]

Originally there could have been little place for love and tenderness; these would emerge very slowly, over thousands of years, and become associated with families and small communities. Survival all the time depended on the rapid and merciless subjection of any opposition, either by animals or by other men, and one imagines that success in these matters would bring a sense of satisfaction and pleasure to the victor and his immediate associates.

There is a tendency to assume that the behaviour of animals is 'instinctive' while our own is the result of learning and thinking. However we sometimes feel that a particular person has a 'cruel streak' or some other hereditary tendency; until recently there was no way of proving this, but now we have direct evidence that certain chromosome distributions in the cell-nucleus (XYY males) predispose to criminal activities, so that one is within sight of identifying the 'born criminal'. This is of course an individual matter, but combined with the coded patterns involved in the behaviour of primitive man we can faintly see some kind of explanation for mass and individual acts of cruelty.

---

[1] *The Identity of Man*, J. Bronowski.
[2] *Man and Technics*, O. Spengler.

Technological and social advances now permit a very large number of men to live, eat and breed without the necessity for overt personal acts of aggression, though some realize that much of their food and clothing is being supplied by the wholesale slaughter of living creatures, often involving much suffering. We are perhaps too close to our ancestors to accept this complete absence of personal violence.

Man's inborn aggressiveness, originally essential for survival, still has a very real function in society, tending to separate the ambitious and successful from the weak and the pig-headed sheep; and without people who get things done in the face of opposition and difficulties we should rapidly decline. Unfortunately frustration in many forms often makes achievement difficult. This begins early in life as discipline of the harshest kind, and continues with bureaucracy, overcrowded roads, boring working conditions and artificial social distinctions. Reaction is seen in children fighting, rough games, enjoyment of fictitious or real violence, idiotic driving and acts of personal spite. Certainly the most primitive and direct form of spite is the infliction of pain. Deep and lasting frustrations derived from oppression will inevitably lead to explosion of these innate aggression tendencies, with mob violence and war. It is significant that the toughest soldiers have always been those most strictly disciplined in training, and allowed release in battle.

Viewed in this light a great many human activities of the kind outlined in Part III perhaps become more understandable. In addition a little comfort may be felt by the innumerable people who are truly horrified by their own uprushes of apparently vicious and spiteful thoughts, sometimes leading to torments of self-recrimination with complex religious and psychiatric reactions. These thoughts arise because we are human beings, because they are memories of our struggle to survive in a hostile world; the very fact that we can recognize them as such, and after looking them in the face reject them in favour of alternatives, should surely make us realize that we are now beginning on another and perhaps more promising evolutionary path – the psycho-social one envisaged by a few modern philosophers. We can also account to some extent for the cruelty exhibited by young children, and for the otherwise ridiculous Christian doctrine of Original Sin. Aggression and cruelty are no longer technical necessities for human progress, but the problems of overcoming them are formidable, and perhaps will prove insuperable. They include shut minds, educational systems forced into political moulds, religions based on deception, government guided by doctrine rather than wisdom, the obvious success of violence, and commerce founded on avarice. Evolution beyond savagery has resulted in the development of higher faculties – the search for knowledge, the exercise of creative skill, the appreciation of beauty and a sense of brotherhood; these seem to have little power against the lurking menace, yet unless this is finally controlled we shall end by destroying ourselves.

The human brain is not a statistical machine that receives information and produces an answer like a computer. The largest operating computers in the world contain about one million units, each capable of a single function – on or off, or something similar. The human body contains a million million cells, and the brain alone has some twenty thousand millions of these, with vast numbers of association fibres. It constantly summates the entire previous experience of the individual, known and forgotten, his genetic background, state of health, emotional condition, the known opinions of others, all known present factors and all known future possibilities; there is probably nothing very exact about any of these fragments of information, but they combine to give an almost instant picture, and this picture can be strongly coloured by impressions that may in fact be completely false. We should ensure that the more subtle factors contributing to this flickering picture are not more distorted than we can help, but this is very difficult, because at any one time there may be several completely conflicting ideas jostling for position, and it takes a rare penetrating quality of thought to find a clear line between them. Most of us have developed the peculiar ability to maintain such contrary opinions in water-tight compartments, rationalizing each at convenient times, a procedure that helps to protect us from going mad; it also enables physicists to become spiritualists, otter-hunters to support animal protection societies, and the devout to burn heretics. This built-in labile inconsistency makes the formulation of any rational system of ethics very difficult indeed.

It may be objected that any system will be useless if we are all savages just below the surface, as bitter facts of the kind presented in this book seem to show. They are nevertheless selected facts, and the majority of people under normal conditions have no conscious wish to hurt or quarrel with their neighbours. Their tendency to do so under powerful leadership does show that deep instincts are easily aroused, and the clear inference is that our leaders should be selected with the very greatest care. The ridiculous ease with which any plausible power-mad psychopath can take over control of groups, unions, parties and entire countries is the kind of atavistic lunacy that needs urgent attention; it will certainly continue so long as rulers spring from political upstarts and the more bombastic members of the armed forces. Whether a country's government is tied up with some particular set of religious beliefs or not can be a good thing or a bad one, certainly the latter if intolerance is a feature. It is a mistake to assume that agnosticism means a rejection of moral values; there are human values that stand higher than blind faith, mental rigidity and crawling servitude. Do you need a God to tell you that cruelty is wrong?

We have looked at a good many human vices: what about the virtues? According to A. J. Ayer[1] these are love and friendship, the pursuit of knowledge, and the creation of works of art. All these categories are open to wide interpretations, some of them anything but virtuous. What is a work of art? A successful and highly regarded modern artist, Francis Bacon, says: 'I think that painting today is pure intuition and luck, and taking advantage of what happens when you splash the bits down.'

It seems almost impossible to define or devise an effective moral code that would guide men away from the innate tendencies and yet leave them to some extent free. Ideally each should give his best, and be encouraged to do so, never causing unnecessary pain. These things can happen in all walks of life, and do not depend on higher education or religious dogma; but such precepts would carry no weight with the dull, the selfish, the resentful, nor with those who consider that everything ought to be provided for them, or who expect ceaseless entertainment without the smallest physical or mental effort on their part. Perhaps certain painful experiences serve to remind us that everything must be paid for by someone, and maybe that a little thought could have avoided the pain.

Many attempts to revise human behaviour are based on the fallacy

[1] In *What I Believe*, a symposium published by Allen & Unwin.

that this can be done by the invention of a new ethic, for example one that welds together a scientific philosophy with art, or literature, or religion. People in the mass (whose behaviour is of vital importance) are not interested in these things except in an extremely superficial way. What views they do have are held with pig-headed obstinacy, yet they can be led like sheep into activities like witch-hunting or Jew-baiting. Religions that have a firm hold on people's minds invariably begin on really young children, and some believe that the good or harm is done by the age of seven years. It seems logical that the only way out of the multitudinous problems of pain is to base early teaching on precepts agreed by men of wisdom, and to place such teaching in the hands of dedicated experts. Beyond this it probably does not matter very much what children believe so long as it is not based on deception and intolerance. The child should not be forced to follow a book of rules or commandments; he must *know* how to conduct himself, particularly in relation to other people or peoples; he must take pride in his own uniqueness, yet recognise his dependence on and obligations to the community; he must learn to look his basic tendencies towards aggression and cruelty in the face, to recognize them and handle them firmly.

It has been said many times that cruelty is the greatest sin — a word with religious connotations. In fact sin is the very bread and butter of religions, for without this concept they could not exist, any more, according to Stekel, than a grocery store could carry on without canned soup. All the great religions have recognized the basic menace of cruelty and tried, not very successfully, to do something about it. Cruelty is deep, instinctive, complex, closely associated with sex and with the will to power. Cruelty and hate are indeed so basic that they have even been regarded as a necessity to us in some form. Freud himself said 'I must have a friend to love and a foe to hate.' This is the thinking behind the theory of *catharsis*, which holds that sadistic literature and shows, with activities like all-in wrestling and bull-fighting, have the effect on those who need it of releasing pent-up aggression and cruelty, leaving the individual purged of them. Modern psychiatric thought does not support this view, neither is it even reasonable. People who take constant purgatives become dependent on them, and develop a morbid interest in defaecation and excreta.

Cruelty feeds and grows on itself to an extent unbelievable unless the facts of warfare, mob violence and persecution are studied. Its coded potentiality lies in wait in the infant, and we have already seen how it is nurtured and encouraged by action and example during childhood, by squalor and callousness, by savage punishments, by indifference to the sufferings of animals, by intolerance, by open derision of 'softness' regarding these matters, and so on. Unless such conditions can be eliminated from a child's environment he has little chance of controlling his naturally aggressive tendencies later in life; yet his individuality and power of self-development must not be repressed unless these are in conflict with the interests and peace of others.

We certainly have to face the necessity to deal with anti-social and criminal activities by individuals or groups, and it is rather important to realize that just because we are able to explain the mechanism behind a person's behaviour this does not necessarily absolve him from responsibility towards his fellows and society. Some kind of action must be taken. It has always been assumed that such action should contain three factors: punishment of the individual; protection of society against him; and discouragement for others to imitate him. The simple, crude and direct method of achieving all this is the *lex talionis*, as old as Man, and still practised. Is the man a thief? Cut off his hand. Rape and murder? Flog him to death. Under such a system you will get little overt crime, but you make cruelty and violence part of life itself. Yet society must protect itself against selfish violent thugs and criminals. Perhaps eventually these tendencies can be educated out, and any offenders will be cured by a combination of ultra-hypnosis and micro-surgical manipulation of chromosomes; until then, even if punishment is considered inappropriate, there must be some deterrent and there must be some protection, so that the majority of people can live in peace.

Man's evolution in the last thousand years or so has taken place mainly in the spheres of communications and social intercourse. It is intensely important for us to be members of a community and to share in its activities, for this is the way we learn to speak our language and perhaps those of others, and fitting into the numerous complexities of modern life. Certain self-styled rebels exhibit their smouldering atavism by increasing outbreaks of hooliganism and mass violence on the slightest pretext; they are very often people intelligent enough to take some interest in affairs other than their own, but infantile in their personal development. They accept spoon-fed welfare and various social conveniences as their rights, but they cry for help quickly enough when in pain.

The solution of these problems can never lie in keeping a child ignorant of the truth or in deliberately deceiving him, yet this is often what happens to those who escape the early cruelty and squalor.

The word education seems to have acquired a narrow, bickering political aroma. The problems of devising and running a system of teaching that will conquer cruelty are formidable indeed, but eventually they will have to be overcome. One can only hope that the future will see teaching as one of the most highly trained and best paid professions in the world, with scrupulous selection and screening of those privileged to guide the young.

Basic aggression can to a large extent be channelled into various competitive games and into conquest of physical and mental problems, but these activities have to be devised with enormous skill if the physically and emotionally weaker are not to be hurt and discouraged. Every child must be made to feel proud of what he can achieve, however little. To curb the brilliant is sheer folly, so is forcing 'education' (as opposed to training) on those totally unfit to receive it.

The difficulty facing us now is that of introducing rational teaching for our children while we ourselves are engaged continually in political, racial, religious and commercial squabbles, with riots and persecution and war active or on the brink of erupting all over the world; and at the same time there can be no end to these miseries until we have universal rational teaching. Perhaps the revision of teaching will come first. If enormous efforts in this direction are successful, I believe a coded genetic pattern could be evolved in time that would take precedence over aggression as an instinctive form of behaviour, so that it would seem obvious to people that they should avoid causing unnecessary pain.

Before this can possibly happen we shall have to know a great deal more about the mechanism of our minds. The more arrogant forms of psychology and psychiatry, which at present are more like religions than sciences, must emerge from their present infantile stage of cloaking ignorance with dogma and obscurantism. They will have to find the basic truth behind every aspect of behaviour, including the epiphenomena of hypnosis and yoga and intense faith.

It is indeed interesting to think about the extent to which people might ultimately be able to control their minds and those of others, based on potentialities known to exist today – even if we confine such speculation to the field of pain.

We found in Part I that although the normal pathways of sensation are fairly regular and distinct the final passage into consciousness is very speculative and variable, and even that pain could be produced without any apparent organic basis at all. The profound modifications of the pain experience caused by threshold and attention variations were also noted. In Part II an experiment was mentioned in which dogs were conditioned to accept burns in order to obtain food, without apparent pain; we also encountered several instances of absent pain in spite of injuries or diseases that normally cause it. The feats of endurance (Part III) include powerful psychological factors, and their operation was discussed in greater detail under Psychotherapy in Part IV.

All these show that under certain very ill-defined circumstances pain can be minimized, or even completely abolished, by an act of will. At the present time this can only be achieved in a rather artificial way, for instance during religious exaltation or with the aid of a trained hypnotist, but once the actual mechanism is understood it should be possible for the normal intelligent human individual quite deliberately to exclude from consciousness any selected part of his incoming stream of sensory impulses – even pain, the most powerful of all. The training necessary to accomplish this would result in the control of any lesser sensations, and hence in the ability to confine attention almost completely on any desired matter, in a way that is now practically the prerogative of genius, greatly facilitating learning processes and the execution of complex tasks. Like any other outstanding ability such powers of concentration might be used for evil as well as good, and one must visualize them combined with the

6

kind of enlightened teaching already tentatively discussed, with a great bias towards understanding and compassion, as opposed to superstition and intolerance.

Initially only a minority of people will acquire powers of this kind, but perhaps these would automatically become the real leaders of men on a world-wide scale; it is difficult to imagine anything more likely to unite the inhabitants of this Earth than a deep understanding of human nature and its problems, and not the least of these problems is that of pain.

Perhaps all this would take a long time, but after all we are very young. Consider our human time-scale against that of all life on earth.

It seems probable that life began on this planet about one thousand million years ago. Suppose we represent this period of time by the twelve hours on the face of a clock, and start the clock at the moment when living cells first appeared. On this scale dinosaurs were roaming the earth seven minutes ago, and Man evolved from his background of primates forty seconds ago. The whole of recorded history occurs in the last half second, and the average man lives a two-thousandth of a second.

Civilization is evidently only just beginning; perhaps the next second or so will be critical.

BIBLIOGRAPHY

ANDREWS, WILLIAM, *Bygone Punishments*. London 1931.

BERG, KARL, *The Sadist*, trans. Olga Illner and George Godwin, London 1938.

BIRCH, RUSSELL, *The Principles of Humane Experimental Technique*. London 1938.

BISHOP, W. J., *The Early History of Surgery*. Oldbourne, London 1960.

BOLITHO, W., *Murder for Profit*. London 1926.

BOSSARD et MAULDE, *Gilles de Rais*, 2me Edition. Paris 1886.

BRAIN, LORD, *Diseases of the Nervous System*. Oxford University Press, 6th Edition. 1962.

BRAMWELL J. MILNE, *Hypnotism*. Rider & Co., London 1930.

BRONOWSKI, J., *The Identity of Man*. Heinemann, London 1966.

BRUNTON, PAUL, *The Hidden Teaching Beyond Yoga*. Rider & Co., London.

CHURCHILL, WINSTON, *Marlborough—His Life and Times*, Vol. I. Harrap, London 1933.

DAWES, CHARLES REGINALD, *The Marquis de Sade, His Life and Works*. Robert Holden, London 1927 (This edition was limited to 100 copies).

DOELL, E. W., *Doctor against Witch Doctor*, Christopher Johnson, 1955.

DOWSETT, J. MOREWOOD, *The Spanish Bull Ring*. J. Bale, London 1928.

DUNLOP, SIR E. and ALSTEAD, STANLEY, *Textbook of Medical Treatment*. E. & S. Livingstone, London 1966.

Encyclopaedia Britannica, 14th edition.

Encyclopaedia of Religion and Ethics. T. & T. Clark, U.S.A. 1909.

EVANS, E. P., *The Criminal Prosecution and Capital Punishment of Animals*. London 1906.

FOX, JOHN, *Acts and Monuments of Martyrs*. 1684.

FRAXI, PISANUS (H. S. Ashbee), *Index Librorum Prohibitorum*, London 1887; *Centuria Librorum Absconditorum*, London 1879; *Catena Librorum Tacendoram*, London 1885.

FRAZER, SIR JAMES, *The Golden Bough* (12 volumes). Macmillan, London 1936.

FRENCH'S *Index of Differential Diagnosis*. John Wright & Sons Ltd, Bristol 1954.

FRITSCH, F. E. and SALISBURY, SIR E., *Plant Form and Function*. Bell, London 1961.

GALLICO, PAUL, *The Hand of Mary Constable*. Heinemann, London 1964.

GALLONI, ANTONIO, *Tortures and Torments of the Christian Martyrs*, Paris 1668; trans. A. R. Allison. London 1903.

GARNETT, HENRY, *Portrait of Guy Fawkes*. Robert Hale, London 1962.

GOULD, G. M., and PYLE, W. L., *Anomalies and Curiosities of Medicine*. W. B. Saunders, U.S.A. 1897.

GRAY, IAN, *Ivan the Terrible*. Hodder & Stoughton. 1964.

GREENWOOD, JAMES, *Curiosities of Savage Life*. London 1863.

HANSFORD JOHNSON, PAMELA, *On Iniquity*. Macmillan, 1967.

HILTON, JOHN, *Rest and Pain*. London 1863; Published by E. Bell & Sons, London 1950.

HOLE, CHRISTINA, *A Mirror of Witchcraft*. Chatto & Windus, 1957.

HUME, C. W., *Man and Beast*. University Federation for Animal Welfare, London 1962.

HUXLEY, ALDOUS, *The Devils of Loudon*. Chatto & Windus, London 1952.

JARDINE, DAVID, *On the Use of Torture in the Criminal Law of England*. 1837.

KARPMAN, B., *The Sexual Offender and his Offences*. Julian Press, New York 1954.

KEIFFER, OTTO, *Sexual Life in Ancient Rome*, trans. G. & H. Highet. G. Routledge & Sons. London 1934.

KNIGHTON, ROBERT S. and DUMKE, PAUL (Editors), *Pain (An International Symposium)*. Henry Ford Hospital, Detroit. Published by Little, Brown & Co., Massachusetts, 1966.

KRAFFT-EBING, R. V., *Psychopathia Sexualis*. Heinemann, London 1931.

KRECKE, ALBERT, *The Doctor and his Patients*. Kegan Paul, London 1934.

LAVINE, EMANUEL H., *The Third Degree*. Vanguard Press, New York 1930.

LEA, HENRY CHARLES, *A History of the Inquisition in Spain*. New York 1906.

,, ,, ,, *A History of the Inquisition in the Middle Ages*. New York 1906.

,, ,, ,, *Superstition and Force*. Philadelphia 1878.

LEWIS, C. S., *The Problem of Pain* (1940). Collins, London 1957.

LEWIS, SIR THOMAS, *Pain*. Macmillan, New York 1942.

LEWISOHN, RICHARD, *Animals Men and Myths*. Gollancz, London 1954.

LICHT, HANS, *Sexual Life in Ancient Greece*. G. Routledge & Sons, London 1931.

MCCABE, JOSEPH, *The Popes and Their Church* (5th Edition). Watts & Co., London 1950.

MANNIX, DAN, *Memoirs of a Sword Swallower*. Hamilton 1951.

MACKAY, CHARLES, *Extraordinary Popular Delusions and the Madness of Crowds*. Re-published by Harrap, London 1956.

MARSHALL, B., *The White Rabbit*. Evans Bros., London 1952.

MELGOUNOV, S. P., *The Red Terror in Russia*. Dent, London 1925.

MALINOWSKI, B., *Sex and Repression in Savage Society*. Kegan Paul, London 1927.

MOORE, PATRICK (Editor), *Against Hunting* (A Symposium). Gollancz, London 1965.

MORRIS, RAMONA AND DESMOND, *Men and Apes*. Hutchinson, London 1966.

New Scientist, October 1967.

OSBORN, ARTHUR W., *The Superphysical*. Nicholson & Watson, London 1937.

Psychosomatic Medicine. The First Hahnemann Symposium. U.S.A. 1962.

RAPER, A. F., *The Tragedy of Lynching*. Chapel Hill, N. Carolina 1933.

REISS, R. A., *Report upon the Atrocities Committed by the Austro-Hungarian Army during the First Invasion of Serbia*; trans. F. S. Copeland. 1916.

RINN, J. F. and HOUDINI HARRY, *Searchlight on Psychical Research*. Rider & Co., U.S.A. 1954.

ROUSSEAU, JEAN JACQUES, *Confessions*. Grant, 1904; Re-published Dent, 1967.

RUSSELL, CLAIRE and RUSSELL, William Moy Stratton, *Human Behaviour*. Deutsch, U.S.A. 1961.

RUSSELL, LORD, *The Scourge of the Swastika*. Corgi Books, London 1954.

SALT, HENRY S., *The Flogging Craze*. London 1916.

SAUERBRUCH, WENKE, *Pain*. German Edition, 1936; George Allen & Unwin, London 1963.

SCOTT, GEORGE RYLEY, *A History of Torture Throughout the Ages*. T. Werner Laurie, London 1940.

SERJEANT, R. B., *Mink on My Shoulder*. Robert Hale, London 1966.

SERJEANT, RICHARD, *A Man May Drink*. Putnam, London 1964.

SIMPSON, KEITH, *The Battered Baby*. 1966.

SPENGLER, O., *Man and Technics*. Allen & Unwin, London 1963.

STEKEL, WILHELM, *Sadism and Masochism*. John Lane, London 1955.

SWAIN, JOHN, *Brutes and Beasts*. Noel Douglas, London 1933.

SUETONIUS, TRANQUILLUS, *The Lives of the Twelve Caesars*. 1717.

TICKELL, JERRARD, *Odette*. Chapman & Hall, London 1956.

TIMPERLEY, H. J., *What War Means; the Japanese Terror in China*. London 1938.

University Federation for Animal Welfare. Handbook. 1966.

VINCENT, A. L. and BINNS, CLARA, *Gilles de Rais*. Philpot, London 1926.

WALSH, SIR CECIL, *Crime in India*. London 1930.

WATSON-JONES, R., *Fractures and Other Bone and Joint Injuries*. E. & S. Livingstone, Edinburgh 1941.

WELLS, LEON, *The Janowska Road*. Jonathan Cape, London.

WESTERLING, RAYMOND, *Challenge to Terror*. Kimber 1952.

What I Believe (Various Authors). Allen & Unwin, London 1966.

WHITE, JAMES C. and SWEET, WILLIAM H., *Pain: Its Mechanism and Surgical Control*. Charles C. Thomas, U.S.A. 1955.

WOLFF, HAROLD G. and WOLF, STEWART, *Pain*. Blackwell, Oxford 1958.

WRIGHT, SAMSON, *Applied Physiology*. Oxford Medical Publications, 1965.

WYLIE, CHURCHILL and DAVIDSON, *A Practice of Anaesthesia*. Lloyd-Luke, U.S.A. 1966.

YOUNG, J. Z., *Doubt and Certainty in Science*. Reith Lectures 1950. Oxford University Press, 1950.

INDEX